Build Your Nest
a postpartum planning workbook

Copyright @ 2021 by Kestrel Gates

All rights reserved. This book or any portion thereof may not be reproduced or used in any manner whatsoever without the express written permission of the author except for the use of brief quotations in a book review, with the exception of the resource pages.

Self Published through Kindle Direct Publishing

First printed 2016
Updated version 2021

The information in this workbook is not meant to diagnose or prescribe.

The workbook is designed and intended to be a single use document.

There is a bulk discount for professionals or groups.

The glossary, Meal Train Guide, Black resource page, and the LGBQT resource page are available for free at **www.buildyournestworkbook.com**

I write with humility knowing that while these words are fixed on the page, science and culture, as well as my personal knowledge and understanding, are always evolving. I also write with certainty that when we are born and when we birth, we will always need love and care. Please do reach out to me with suggestions, feedback, ideas, and feelings.

Hello dear reader,

The postpartum time is like none other in our lives.

It is a time to surrender to our most wild animal-self, the ferocity and the tenderness, for within this lies our deepest need to mother.

It is a time for slowing down, taking joy in our precious newborn, and feeling held by our circles of support.

It can be sweet and simple.

My hope is that your planning will set you up for a joy-filled postpartum time.

And that you come through transformed and triumphant.

With love,

~Kestrel

Table of Contents

Postpartum
- 7   How Long?
- 9   Recovery Experiences
- 10   In the Water
- 11   3 Tools
- 12   Your Vision
- 13   Lineage Traditions

Your People
- 16   Partner
- 19   Solo Mama
- 20   Your Circles
- 28   Doulas

Preparing
- 29   Rest
- 33   Feeding Your Baby
- 38   Nourishment
- 39   Health
- 44   Mental Health
- 46   Home
- 48   Family
- 51   Money
- 54   Back to Work

Recovery Extenders
- 56   The Unexpected
- 57   Back to Basics
- 58   Cesarean Recovery
- 62   NICU
- 64   Multiples

The Plan
- 67   Milk Retreat
- 68   Postpartum Net
- 69   Your People
- 71   The Plan
- 77   Budget
- 78   Calendar

Appendix
- 83   Pregnancy-To-Do-List
- 84   Help!
- 85   Birth Considerations
- 86   Resources*
- 89   Glossary*
- 96   Meal Train Guide*

Available on-line as a free download at: www.buildyournestworkbook.com

There is no one right way!

DO IT YOUR WAY

This workbook is set up to encourage you to get creative with your set of circumstances.

It sometimes happens that after we give birth we have all the time and the support needed to fully recover and joyfully bond with our newborn

Welcome — how to use this workbook

My intention is to support you in having the best possible postpartum experience.

Give yourself permission to dream up a vision for this time with your newborn. Allow this vision to act as your compass, guiding you. Ask for what you need, draw boundaries when you want them. Claim this precious time and fill it with love.

This workbook is designed to be worked with during pregnancy, however it can be used after the baby is born as well. If your baby has been born, you may wish to start by reading page 80. I have included more ideas than you can possibly do. These are not meant to be to-do lists! Pick and choose what makes sense for you and your family and add in your own ideas as well.

By the end, I hope you have a pregnancy to-do list, clear plans for getting your needs met, a strong circle of support in place, a specific plan for taking time off and resource list that will be there for any unexpected challenges.

My suggestion for creating your plan is this:

1. Give the entire Workbook a light reading, then sleep on it and allow some time to pass

2. Go back through and write in your answers to the questions. Circle and star ideas and concepts that you are drawn to. Add your own ideas. Mark it up; make it yours. (It may be nice to use a pencil so that you can adjust as your ideas change.) Cross out the ideas that you don't like or that aren't feasible.

3. Allow some time to pass, and then come back to it and use the plan template in the back, refining it as you discuss it with your key support people

Bring your partner or primary support people into the process as feels right. Allow time for brainstorming sessions and dialogues so that, as you get the details worked out, your closest people are on board. Maybe you and your partner take turns reading it out loud, or maybe you each write down answers to questions separately and then discuss. It is worth experimenting to find creative ways to make the planning process collaborative and fun.

With this workbook, you will find that my focus is primarily on you, the person who has just given birth, and not on the baby. This is because I believe that when you are well supported, caring for the baby becomes much easier as your inner wisdom and natural instincts are strengthened. And with a resource list in place, you will know whom to call when questions do come up. I also see tremendous value in centering mothers experiences and following their desires to meet their babies' needs without layering her up with parenting "shoulds". That said, it can be so helpful to find friends and care providers that share similar parenting philosophies from whom to learn and draw inspiration.

There are so many ways that families are formed. I use both the words "mother" and "birthing /postpartum person/people" to be inclusive of all identities, while also recognizing that by in large readers of this workbook will be people who identify as woman and mother. Throughout the workbook I refer to the reader as "you" or "we" so as to not assume your gender identity. I use the terms "partner" and "they" to be inclusive of all types of relationships and identities and genders.

Also, know that I am not a mental health or medical professional. Please seek professional support when needed. In the appendix you will find the Glossary of Postpartum Terms and also the Meal Train Guide. These are free resources available on my website. The Meal Train Guide is for sharing with someone else who will organize your Meal Train.

There is no one right way!

This is not a to-do list or a cookie cutter plan.
Cross out the ideas that you don't like or truly aren't feasible!
Write down your own ideas.

Cultural shift, one family at a time!

A postpartum plan

A postpartum plan is an outline of how you will get the rest, support, and care you need after your baby is born. It is specific to you, your family, and your set of circumstances.

There are two main aspects of the plan.
The "Milk Retreat" is a set amount of time for rest, support, and care. I call this a "Milk Retreat" because during these early weeks with newborns so much time is spent feeding the baby. With so much going on physically and psychologically it makes sense to have a period of time that is set aside from normal life -a retreat.

The "Postpartum Net" is the contingency part of the plan that details resources for unexpected challenges and plans for extending the time of rest and support. Deciding that you are going to call a specific person in the case that, for example, breastfeeding is hard, makes it much more likely that you will reach out and get support.

The "Milk Retreat" can look a lot of different ways. Maybe your own mother comes to be with you for the first month. Maybe you hire a postpartum doula. Maybe you have complete support for the first week. Maybe you stay home, with only a few exceptions, for the first 6 weeks. Maybe you have a few close friends who agree to come regularly and spend big blocks of time with you during the first weeks. Maybe you are following your culture of origin's traditional protocols.

I am outlining what all mothers, all birthing people and their families deserve. Going through this workbook will look really different for different people. It is important to keep in mind that even the best made plan will not protect a family from feeling the effects of a culture that doesn't support families. The idea that rest, support, and care after giving birth are basic human rights, does not fit the economic and social realities of the U.S. We need change throughout our society, from the internalized pressure that mothers face, all the way up to the national level, granting paid parental leave. This is a cultural shift. By finding ways to have rest and support during the postpartum period we are engaging in this shift. There are also systemic racial inequities that affect birth and postpartum experiences. This too is being addressed within communities, and in the state and national political spheres. Eventually, if you are interested in getting involved at a structural level there are many organizations to connect with. Moms Rising (www.mothersrising.org) is an example of a national organization that addresses many important issues. For now, you can give yourself permission to focus on your family and on your own wellbeing.

Sometimes the biggest blocks to having rest, support, and care are the ways that the culture affects our thinking and feeling. We may feel pressure to prove ourselves as the mythological "good mothers". Or we may be thinking that because mothering is "natural" it must be easy. Or we don't want to bother anyone with our needs. Or that because we wanted this baby so badly we shouldn't express our need for help if we are having a hard time. Parenting is a path of personal cultivation, meaning that it pushes us to grow. It takes us to our core, touches on our deepest wounds, giving us an opportunity for tremendous growth. Mothering transforms us.

This is your journey.

I hope this workbook can help you on your way.

~ Kestrel

Some say postpartum lasts as long as your child is in diapers, breastfeeding, and not sleeping through the night!

How Long?

The postpartum period is the time after birth when the new mother is recovering physically and emotionally from pregnancy and birth, and integrating her new role as mother to her baby. The duration of recovery and adjustment is individual, though often takes a full year. Medically the postpartum period is viewed as six weeks, however many complications have not yet been resolved or even begun by six weeks. Common examples are complications with breastfeeding, pelvic floor issues, and mental health issues.

My recommendation is to set up a "Milk Retreat" so that you have a specific time period that is designated for recovery and bonding, with the understanding that you very well may be continuing to recover in the weeks and months to follow. Four to six full weeks of rest and care is common around the world and this is a good basic time frame to plan for, if there aren't any complications. For some people this isn't possible because they need to go back to work or don't have the support networks needed. Give yourself as much time as you can get.

Each family is different and their postpartum plan will need to reflect their individual preferences, needs, and resources. A few ways families are different are finances, familial support, community, and employment. The key to working with limitations is being able to see where you can ask for more time or more support. Keep an open mind and get creative.

If you live in the United States, consider that we generally have much less time for recovery and bonding than almost anywhere in the world. The United States is one of nine countries that doesn't offer maternity leave -the other 8 are small and undeveloped. In contrast, Canada gives mothers 50 weeks!

Parenting a newborn is big, important, and often challenging work, and mothers absolutely deserve to be fully supported in their physical recovery and their emotional adjustment to parenting a new baby. This is true for the first baby as much as it is for each subsequent birth.

While the focus of this workbook is the first weeks and months after your baby's birth, these resources and concepts may help you meet challenges that arise later on as well. Postpartum depression and struggles with breastfeeding are examples of issues that can happen through the toddler years that may deserve professional help and slowing down.

Wow, is there a lot going on!

Recovery experiences

Along with having a darling baby, we have so much going on with our bodies, our hearts, and our spirits. We are transitioning out of being pregnant, recovering from birth, bonding with, and learning to care for a newborn, and breastfeeding. We may be parenting older children as well. The following three lists may put in perspective why rest, support, and care are so needed. "Many" is for anything that happens for at least 1 out of 4 people after birth. And "Some" is 1 out of 5 people or more. These are rough estimates. This is information to share with partners and close support people. It is not meant to normalize or minimize the impact of these experiences. Reach out and get the emotional, practical, and medical support you need. Do not suffer in silence!

Everyone	Many	Some
• Healing in the pelvic bowl (bones, muscles, organs, tissues of the pelvis) • 3-6 weeks of lochia, vaginal bleeding • All body systems adjusting to not being pregnant • All body systems adjusting to breastfeeding • Sleep deprivation, interrupted sleep • Milk comes in at 2-4 days after birth	• Aching muscles • Painful "after-pains" (contractions to shrink uterus) • Healing from tears, vaginal skin abrasions or "skid marks" • Healing from episiotomy • Hemorrhoids, anal fissures • Constipation • Loose bowel movements • Pain with peeing and pooping • Low grade fever on day 3 or 4 • Chills and shakes • Huge range of emotions • Weepiness • Irritability • Disturbing day/night dreams (invasive thoughts) • Overwhelm • Anxiety • Fear • Sore nipples • Cracked nipples • Thrush (yeast on nipples or baby's mouth) • Mother and baby both learning to nurse • Spraying or leaking breasts • Breast engorgement • Recovery from Cesarean birth • Aftermath of a traumatic birth • Perinatal mood and anxiety disorders symptoms: extreme mental states (PMAD)	• Extreme pain with nursing • Pain with let down • Significant trouble nursing • Mastitis-breast infection • Insufficient milk • Serious pelvic issues • Uterine infection • Extended hospital stay • Time in neonatal intensive care unit (NICU) • Multiple babies • Premature baby • Incontinence • Pubic symphysis • Diastasis recti • PMAD's: perinatal mood and anxiety disorders, including depression, anxiety, Obsessive, Compulsive Disorder (OCD), psychosis • Post traumatic stress disorder (PTSD) • Bonding difficulties

In the water

These phases are not medical or biological. They are a subjective way of seeing the postpartum period and may be helpful for planning. You may jump from the "Flotation Device" to "Swimming" during your first week, then find your self back to the "Doggy Paddle" when your partner goes back to work or your mother goes home. Or it might not be until your baby is 8 months old that you feel like you are "Swimming". The key here is to allow for rest and support to continue even if you are "Swimming".

Flotation Device

You are still at the hospital or birth center, or your homebirth midwives are still at your house. You are receiving medical attention and are being completely taken care of. Your baby may be cared for by medical staff and may be in the NICU. There can be a sense that things are happening TO you and your baby. This can feel safe and supportive, or it can also feel disorienting and disrespectful.

Doggy Paddle

Your family is now on its own. You are home from the hospital. You may feel overwhelmed as you juggle all the elements of baby care, recovery, and home life.

Fully Swimming

Your family has coordinated breath and movement. You have a sense of having "figured it out". Sleeping and eating rhythms begin to take their form and your family finds its new normal. There is an overall sense of confidence with meeting future challenges. Of course, parenting continues to stretch our capacities as our children grow and develop and unchartered waters can send us back into a sense of doggie paddling.

You have permission to ask for help, to have boundaries, and to slow down!

3 Tools

The Loudspeaker

is a call for help. It is our right and responsibility to speak up when we need help from our health care team, our partners, and our communities. Sometimes we must pass the loudspeaker to a doula or a partner or a friend and let them get help for us. This is not a time to suffer quietly! It is a time to feel seen, heard, and be taken care of.

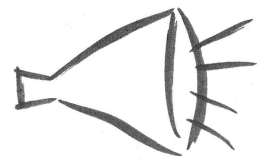

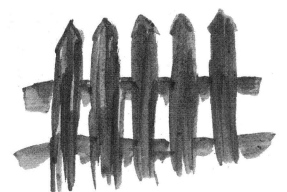

The White Picket Fence

is a boundary. We get to say "no thank you" or "I can't" or simply "No." This comes in handy with unwanted procedures, unwanted guests or visitors, volunteer positions, non-urgent responsibilities, and negativity in any form.

The Slow Down Dial

is a reminder that we can choose to slow life down, even a little. When challenges arise and the overall family stress level goes up, it is probably time to slow down. Maybe you get some help or maybe you are able to back out of some of your responsibilities. You don't have to do everything. In fact, you cannot, and that's O.K.

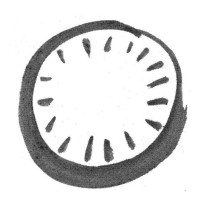

you do you

Your vision ~ Your Compass

What is your vision for the time after your baby is born? Fill this page with writing, allowing all your ideas and images to pour out. How do you want to feel? How do you want your house to be? Who do you want around? What do you want to be doing? What is the over all tone of the experience you dream of? Explore any fears that are coming up. What are you worried about? Then read through what you have written and circle 1-3 words or phrases that stand out as the most important. Maybe you are focussing on a general feeling like "peaceful" or maybe you are focussing on a specific aspect like breastfeeding. Write these in the box below and let this be a compass to guide you. Your postpartum planning process can be guided by this vision and during your postpartum time you can use this to help you make decisions. It is not a guarantee, it is a compass to help you navigate your way.

talk to your grandmothers, your aunties, your mother

Lineage

Giving birth to the next generation connects us in a new way to the generations that have come before us, our lineage. Pregnancy, birth, and postpartum are largely physiological, and yet, how we navigate this childbearing time is highly cultural.

In the United States, the prevailing culture does not recognize that after giving birth we need to be cared for. We are affected by the medicalization of the process and the economic push to return to the workforce. Most people don't feel connected to their own lineage traditions. There are, however, many communities who are both continuing and revisiting their ancestral traditions.

There are two reasons that I am an advocate for continuing postpartum traditions. First, doing so can strengthen our ties to our living family, our ancestors, and cultures of origin. And second, there is a profound wisdom in postpartum traditions that addresses needs for recovery, and our capacity to care for newborns. That said, for people who do have the support of their families, it can be a delicate balance of honoring family and following one's own truth. In other words, for some people the pressure to follow traditions doesn't feel good.

For families who feel bereft of postpartum traditions, you may be able to uncover traditions you weren't aware of by asking older family members or by researching your cultures of origin. Additionally, there is a free, public project that collates postpartum traditions at www.m2mpostpartum.org.

As you work through the workbook and make your postpartum plan, see where you can integrate your lineage's postpartum traditions. And if you feel like you are starting from scratch, imagine you are nurturing traditions that can be passed down, renewing your own ancestral line.

the unity and diversity of humanity

Postpartum Traditions

All of our ancestors had cultural practices to address the needs of the postpartum time. Most people alive today face significant disruptions of these traditions - whether it happened hundreds of years ago or is ongoing. These disruptions have come in many forms. Some of them are: colonization, war, immigration, slavery, religious upheaval, cultural assimilation, diminished value of women, medicalization, and changing economic systems. Cultural trauma and many cultural changes affect postpartum care. What this means is that we relate to our own postpartum lineage traditions in many different ways.

As the scientific fields of human development, neuroscience, nutrition, psychology etcetera, continue to advance, the science is showing that there is tremendous wisdom in so many of the postpartum traditions. There is wisdom in, and evidence for, feeding us nourishing foods, keeping us warm, allowing us to rest and recover, applying herbs and healing touch. The story that this type of care is backwards and unnecessary, is proving to be a myth that is damaging at both personal and cultural levels.

The following page shows some universal elements of postpartum care and speaks to a few specific cultural practices. Some of these practices are alive and well within the culture they originated, others are nearly forgotten, and still others are dying out within their original context, but are continued by other people. Some of us are fortunate to have access to traditional care from within our families. When this knowledge isn't readily available, people may craft a do-it-yourself approach, combined with hiring professionals who hold the knowledge.

All this said, I hope that awareness and care are given when incorporating traditions that are not of one's own lineage. Some traditions are shared freely, while others are withheld and guarded as sacred.

The following list is not intended to be a comprehensive look at traditional practices, but rather an overview that can give readers a sense of both the diversity and the universal nature of these traditions. Other elements that aren't included are rituals of celebration, healing touch, baby care, and the various types of care attendants.

the unity and diversity of humanity

Postpartum Traditions

rest period
A rest period is a specified amount of time devoted to caring for the mother. Much of Africa, Europe, the Middle East, and Latin America have a tradition of forty days. An example is la cuarentena from Latin America, which comes from the word cuarenta meaning forty. In East Asia thirty days are common, as in "sitting the month" in China. In the Hopi tradition rest period is 20 days. In Nigeria, mother and baby traditionally stay in seclusion for 2-3 months. In Vietnam, traditionally a new mother would spend the first three months with her own parents in order to be cared for. This return to one's parents has been practiced in other cultures as well and correlates with
a longer period of rest.

nourishing foods
While diet varies greatly throughout the world, the practice of feeding new mothers nourishing meals that are warming and easily digestible, often including galactogogues to support milk production, is universal. Invariably, foods served during the postpartum time are thoroughly cooked, served warm, and are heavily spiced. Examples of this include soups, porridges and hot drinks. In Korea, there is the seaweed soup called miyeok guk. In Nigeria there is a peanut and rice porridge. In Scandinavia there is also a rice porridge. In the Netherlands, there is an anise seed biscuit. A sweet anise tea is served in Lebanon.

warmth
Keeping new mothers warm is universal and so many traditions work to accomplish this. This includes staying out of the cold weather, avoiding cold or cooling foods, and adding warmth or heat. There is the South East Asian tradition of placing coals under the mother's bed. In Finland mothers would give birth and have their postpartum recovery time in the sauna.

belly wrapping
Belly wrapping is warming and supportive and can be as simple as wrapping a piece of cloth around the belly. There are specific types of wrapping like the interweaving wrapping of the Malaysian style of bengkung and a similar method has been done in Cuba. Germanic peoples had their own way of wrapping, and in Mexico there is the faja. The use of a shawl, or now commonly referred to as rebozo, for healing and ceremony are used in Mexico, Russia and Morocco.

vaginal steaming and sitz baths
Sitz baths are a shallow herbal bath that a person sits in. They are used in European folk medicine, as well as the Caribbean. Vaginal or pelvic steaming is traditional to every continent; to name a few places: Mexico, Malaysia, Italy, Morocco, Korea, Lakota Nation, Haiti, and Korea. Both practices provide warmth and the healing properties of herbs. Sitz baths are gentle and present very little risk. Vaginal steaming offers powerful healing, deeper heat, and a uterine cleanse, but must be practiced safely, with knowledge and care.

different roles, same team

Partner

Your partner, if you have one, is also profoundly affected by a new baby. They too, have needs for support, rest, and appreciation. They too need a recovery time after the birth, especially if it was traumatic for them in any way. If they were worried for your or your baby's life they may suffer from postpartum traumatic stress or PTSD. It is important to remember that the partner is now expected to take on a role that traditionally has been filled by many female relatives. This is just another reason for building a strong circle of support. We also must acknowledge that our relationship is forever transformed with the birth of each child.

While it is obvious, it is worth stating that our roles as partners in parenting newborns are very different, likewise, our experiences of birth and recovery. It is very important for the partner to have an understanding of the postpartum time and the needs of a newborn and a new mother. That said, given our over-all cultural neglect of the postpartum time, it may be hard for a partner to fully understand.

Sometimes there is a concern that a partner is not bonding enough with the baby, especially for exclusively breastfed babies. It can be helpful to remember that there are many ways in addition to feeding to bond, and that bonding happens over a long period of time.

How a partner can help:

- Help keep food and fluids near
- Give emotional and physical support
- Act as a buffer between you and unsupportive family members or friends
- Help link you to the support and information you need
- Minimize their own non-essential wishes and desires (for the initial postpartum period)
- Be flexible about sleeping arrangements

Our Stories
"We came up with a plan — I took care of everything that went into our baby (breastfeeding) and she took care of everything that came out!"

different roles, same team

Partner

The birth of a baby changes a relationship in profound ways. It has the potential to strengthen a couple's bond, and it can take a significant toll. For some couples the changes to their sexual intimacy is particularly challenging. The key here is that there isn't a set timeline of when or how this will play out. Being ready for sex after birth is completely individual, it's about our own desire for sex, and not a medical check up at six weeks. While so much focus is on recovery and on the baby, it is important to tend to your relationship as well. Here are some questions to help you tend to your relationship before your baby comes.

What are current sources of stress in your relationship?

What nourishes your relationship? How do you enjoy spending time together?

Here are some ideas to consider: (you can add more ideas below)

- Work on expected disagreements ahead of time, while you are still pregnant
- Discuss your parenting philosophies
- Have the name of a recommended couples therapist, minister, or friend ally
- Don't expect things to be "fair" or "equal" -accept your different roles in parenting a baby
- Your partner needs rest and time to bond as well
- Eventually claim one night a week to be "date night" -this can be just snuggling on the couch while the baby sleeps
- Remember to express love and appreciation
- Continue to talk about your individual needs for sexual intimacy and find patience for the changes a baby can have on this

Your People

different roles, same team

Partner

This is for you and your partner to work on together.
This is an opportunity for you each to talk about your expectations, needs, and wishes. It is a time to take a really close look at their responsibilities in the home and away. It is not about figuring out how the two of you can do it all on your own. It is about seeing where you may need additional support. It may be helpful to put anything related to time on the calendar.

How long do they have off from work? Is there some wiggle room to make this longer if unexpected challenges arise with postpartum?

What responsibilities around the house are they already doing?

What added responsibilities will they take on and for how long?

If there are older children, what parenting responsibilities are they already doing?

What responsibilities will they take on and for how long?

How do you plan to keep stress low and support connection?

What can they do for their own stress relief and support?

calling in your community

Solo Mama

A well supported postpartum time without a partner may require considerable planning during pregnancy. Take time and attention to solidify your relationships, building your circle of support. Identify the help you need and know that you may need to rely on many people. And be flexible, knowing that change will happen in your support circles: some people won't be available and others will step in. Plan for as much support as you can.

Here are some ideas to consider: (you can add more ideas below)

- Get as much maternity leave as possible
- Ask friends and family to contribute money to a postpartum fund
- Plan to have someone there with you around the clock for at least the first week
- Then plan on someone to come over so that you can take showers and have your hands free. See "mama-sitter" in the glossary
- Organize long term meal planning and housecleaning support
- Consider hiring a postpartum doula, some doula training programs provide student doulas at low or no cost

families come in all shapes and sizes

Your Circles family

Each family is truly unique. Families vary in all sorts of ways: size, gender, location, emotional dynamics, history, cultural make-up, finances, work life, pace of life, communication, values . . . etc!

All of this comes into play with postpartum planning and parenting in general.

Bringing awareness to the specifics of your family make-up may help with planning for the postpartum.

Maybe your partner can't get any time off from work.
Maybe your sister lives across the street and is very supportive.
Maybe your in-laws have very different parenting ideas than you.

These are the type of factors that will affect how you plan. They aren't things that you can change, they are things to accept and work with.

What are some factors that may be challenging?

What are some factors that may be helpful?

some research shows that having a strong sense of community may be a factor that has greater impact on our health than nutrition and exercise

Your Circles concentric rings of support

In this section, write down as many people and resources as you can think of and come back to these lists when making your postpartum plan. Allow your postpartum to be a time of receiving support, and know that you will have so many opportunities in the future to reciprocate

Make a list of all the people in your life who will support you.

Whether it is your best friend on the other side of the country who just loves you; or your neighbor who will watch your older kids; or your mother who won't be cooking for you, but will be doing all the laundry and greeting visitors; your old co-worker who will bring a meal by; or whether your church group who will bring you supplies, or your acupuncturist who will help return the heat to your body. Imagine that there are concentric circles of support around you. Write down everyone you can think of!

Your People

some research shows that having a strong sense of community may be a factor that has greater impact on our health than nutrition and exercise

Your Circles personal, free, paid

Within a postpartum circle of support there are friends and family, free resources, and paid professional resources. With this in mind make three lists -which may or may not overlap with the brainstorm from the previous page. As you work through the workbook keep adding to these lists.

Friends and family who will support you in any way:

Free resources online and in person, including all that your insurance covers:

Professionals that are paid out of pocket:

some research shows that having a strong sense of community may be a factor that has greater impact on our health than nutrition and exercise

Your Circles inner circle

Within these concentric circles of support there is an inner circle. You can include your partner as part of your inner circle or place your partner with you in the center. And more than just thinking of whom you are close with, but who has time and or emotional energy to offer the support you may need during postpartum. Know that sometimes people we expect to be supportive are not able to and that in their place other people step forward. Be flexible.

Consider setting up an "A-team" which is two to four friends who have agreed to be your allies, aunties, and advocates. This is a way of bringing intentionality to friendship so that the friends can work together in providing support.

Make a list of your close people and how they will help.

some research shows that having a strong sense of community may be a factor that has greater impact on our health than nutrition and exercise

Your Circles network of parents

One of the biggest sources of support for mothers of babies is their network of other mothers or parents. Often this network must be built over time with intention and effort. And for many people, this network includes real time friends as well as an on-line component. These other mothers can be an invaluable source of parenting information and support. For queer and trans / nonbinary folks finding parents you relate to is essential.

Here are some ideas to consider: (you can add more ideas below)

- Find groups that meet up regularly, many of which can be joined during pregnancy: free postpartum groups, La Leche League meetings, stroller or babywearing walking groups
- Take a class during pregnancy: childbirth education, breastfeeding, yoga, etc
- Reach out to other mothers in your neighborhood and find a walking buddy
- Connect with local parents through social media groups
- Connect with mothers through social media groups that focus on a specific philosophy or parenting practice

Who are you already connected to?

Who do you want to reach out to?

What are some ways you will build your network?

sweet connection and good boundaries

Your Circles visitors

Having visitors can be wonderful and it can also be exhausting. Some people come to help and are sensitive to the needs of a family with a newborn. Other people come and just want to visit. In these pages explore who you are expecting to visit and how you would like to include them in your circle of support and/or what boundaries you would like to have.

Make a list below of drop-in visitors as well as people coming from out of town. Consider how you feel about each person. Does this person nourish or take away from your overall sense of well-being? What can they help with or what boundary would you like to draw?

Your People

sweet connection and good boundaries

Your Circles visitors

Here are some possible boundaries to consider: (you can add more ideas below)

- Set and share that you are available for a limited time, such as 15 minutes
- Simply excuse yourself or say that you need to rest when you are tired out
- Do not be a hostess in any way
- Ask visitors to wash their hands -have a sign up or someone else to ask
- No one has to hold your baby
- Visitors can be asked to help
- Out of town family can be invited to visit after a certain number of days or weeks
- Out of town family can stay with you or somewhere else
- Put a to-do list on the wall of jobs visitors can choose from
- Be ready to cancel if you aren't up for having visitors
- Set up visiting hours
- Create a family quarantine sign to use when you are not up for visits at a short notice

some research shows that having a strong sense of community may be a factor that has greater health implications than nutrition and exercise

Your Circles asking for help

One of the biggest barriers to having the support you need is asking for help. Many people feel honored to be involved in supporting a family of a newborn. Others have been on the receiving end of this type of support and know how valuable it is and are delighted to get to return the favor. And there are some people who don't understand and won't participate. Or some that do understand but are unable for various reasons to help.

It is worth asking. Know that there will be so many opportunities in the future to reciprocate this support. It is by giving and receiving that we cultivate community in our lives. The community that you foster when your baby is born, may enrich your child's life. Know that you deserve support beyond the time you are struggling (in "doggy paddle" phase) into when you are feeling more recovered and in the flow (the "fully swimming phase").

As much as you can get your partner, close support people, and extended community to understand your plan and why it is needed the more support you will have.

Here are some ways of asking for help to consider: (you can add more ideas below)

- Put someone else in charge of asking. If you are planning on having a meal train, have someone else organize it for you. This person can let people know what you need and when, which takes away the awkwardness of asking for yourself. Someone else can also be in charge of your "kid Train" or your cleaning, or gift registry as well.

- Specific people for specific jobs. Make a list of specific ways that you need help and then think of the right people for each job and ask them individually. Someone comes by to take care of your garden, someone organizes your meal Train, and someone takes your kids on a weekly date.

- Use your baby shower as an easy way to get people organized and on board. In the process of being invited to your baby shower or mama blessing, guests can be encouraged to join in on helping. Or once people are gathered. It can be a wonderful time for a clipboard sign up sheet to be passed around for people to sign-up.

- Gifts. Get specific with what you need. Maybe you really do need some baby supplies and you make a registry for this. Maybe you have your supplies and you ask people to donate their time with bringing meals and cleaning. Or maybe you ask for donations of any amount to go towards your postpartum doula and diaper service.

doula = mothering the mother

Doulas

The support of doulas is invaluable. There is a huge body of research showing that the presence of a doula can improve birth and breastfeeding outcomes. Families benefit in so many ways from having this knowledgeable support as part of their birth and postpartum plans. With most people living far from their families or challenged by emotional or philosophical distances, a doula can help fill this void.

There are two main types of doulas: the birth doula and the postpartum doula.

A birth doula is a trained labor assistant who tends to mothers during labor and delivery. She provides continuous emotional support, as well as assistance with other non-medical aspects of care, and can help navigate the plethora of medical choices that may arise.

A postpartum doula provides support and guidance to a new mother and her family. She offers guidance in breastfeeding and newborn care. She does light household chores, meal preparation, errands, and care of mother and baby. A postpartum doula's care is catered to the family's needs.

There are also "full spectrum doulas" who provide support to families through all pregnancy experiences, including birth, abortion, adoption, surrogacy, miscarriage and stillbirth.

With planning and communication, the support of a doula can be woven into the larger fabric of your support network. This may look like hiring a birth doula and having your partner prepare to support you through labor by attending child birth education class. Or it may look like having your mother-in-law come, receiving a Meal Train, and hiring a postpartum doula. Including doulas in your birth and postpartum plans strengthens your plans immeasurably. Doulas do not replace the need for a plan.

Doulas are worth their weight in gold. They are worth adjusting your budget for. If you truly don't have the funds, there may be doulas who are in training or take clients on a sliding scale basis. Or friends and family can contribute to a doula fund for a baby shower gift.

We call it "rest" but really it is a lot of work (and not much sleep) caring for a newborn and fully recovering!

Rest how long?

It is very helpful to set a time frame for how long you plan on having to rest. If your family or culture of origin has a tradition around this it may be meaningful and helpful to simply follow this time line. Examples of traditional postpartum times are in Mexico forty days, "La Cuarentena", and in China, thirty days or "Zuo Yue Zi". For people who are not connected to their lineage postpartum practices, I have coined the term "Milk Retreat" which is a set amount of time a mother chooses to receive nourishing food, warmth, rest, and special care in order to fully recover from birth.

Rest is the most important factor for healing and recovery. Without rest your body is a bit like a leaky bucket and the impact of every thing else you do to support recovery is weakened. What a postpartum person is actually doing while resting is huge: caring for a newborn around the clock, feeding the baby, recovering from pregnancy and birth, and surfing huge hormonal waves and big emotions. Postpartum mothers need rest. Having time to rest lowers stress which is hugely beneficial for newborns whose state of being is inseparable from their mothers. Further more, this time of rest allows for bonding that supports the wellbeing of both mother and baby.

In families and cultures with postpartum traditions in place, and in some European healthcare systems, postpartum care happens to mothers.

It is not enough to agree with the *idea* of resting after your baby is born. You need a time-line with specifics that detail what you are resting from. You need this agreement with yourself so that any inner critical voices that crop up can be quieted. Plan this out ahead of time so that you can arrange for the support needed to make it possible. You can't simply say you will not do any dishes for 3 weeks.
You need to ask someone else to step in, and you need to be able to give them a concrete time frame.

How long is your Milk Retreat? How many weeks?

Then, revisit this after working through the following pages and come up with your answer.

Notice what feelings come up when you imagine resting for that long. Jot these down.

Preparing

Our Stories

"Newborns have a way of taking over! I thought I could just strap her on and keep going. But then it all caught up with me and I learned that I needed to rest. That mothering this tiny person really is a lot of work in and of its self."

We call it "rest" but really it is a lot of work (and not much sleep) caring for a newborn and fully recovering!

Rest time off

List your current responsibilities and activities.

What are your current responsibilities in your home, your work, your community? If you are self-employed it is helpful to list your roles and responsibilities separately. Next to each responsibility you listed below, write down how long you would ideally take off. Revisit this and come up with your final plan.

household

paid work

personal pursuits

social

volunteering

We call it "rest" but really it is a lot of work (and not much sleep) caring for a newborn and fully recovering!

Rest time off

Here are some ideas that support rest: (you can add more ideas below)

- Delegate household duties

- Avoid news or other sources of negativity

- Be out of touch, socially -including any and all on-line platforms. Set up an automated email response explaining you are on maternity leave and will be back in touch soon

- Make a specific plan about your phone use. Scrolling is not actually resting, nor does it support bonding

- Have someone in charge of your "postpartum PR" and make sure that they are telling your story right. This becomes especially important when facing any extended postpartum circumstances, such as time in the NICU, cesarean recovery, or PMAD's. It can be helpful to have someone else there to communicate how you are doing and what you are needing. This can be your birth announcements, blog posts, social media, or emailing your meal train people etc

- If possible, avoid other life transitions, such as moving, changing jobs, big house improvements, getting new pets, etc

We call it "rest" but really it is a lot of work (and not much sleep) caring for a newborn and fully recovering!

Rest staying in

Staying home is an important aspect of resting. It is much easier to focus on our own recovery, our baby's needs, and on establishing a breastfeeding relationship in the comfort of our own homes. Some people need privacy for feeding their babies, and may feed their babies less when they are out and about. If staying home sounds really unappealing, I encourage you to set a time frame for staying home and then when you do leave your house, only do it for activities that are absolutely necessary or activities that you feel nourished by. Think about other places that feel like home. The idea of staying home is not to set you up for being "bad at staying home" or a "failure" if you do leave. It is about prioritizing being at home and putting your needs first. There are many ways to address the solitude that many mothers face at home. A Meal Train can be a way to have a schedule of visitors in place. Or having a "mama sitter," a friend who comes over to spend time with you, so that you are not alone with your baby (and older siblings).

Consider the following ideas for staying in: (you can add more ideas below)

- Stay inside
- Stay home
- Stay in bed or on the couch
- Keep warm and avoid the cold and the wind
- Stay in pajamas or other comfy lounge wear
- The first time you leave the house, do something enjoyable and for no more than one hour
- Prioritize professionals (IBCLC, body workers, etc) who do home visits
- If you had hospital prenatal care and birth, you may be able to find a homebirth midwife to provide in home postpartum and well baby care
- Have a someone accompany you to your outings

Our Stories
"Even though it was hard for me I really took my midwives' advice to heart: 2 weeks in bed, 2 weeks on the bed, and 2 weeks near the bed".

breastfeeding —natural but not necessarily easy!

Feeding Your Baby

For some parent-baby pairs, feeding comes easily. For others huge challenges arise. If you experience any issues, it is worth getting the support you need as soon as possible. Waiting exacerbates most issues. Please, know ahead of time who you will call for help.

During the first few weeks a mother and baby are establishing their breastfeeding relationship. Having a set period of rest or a "Milk Retreat" supports this process. Because in the womb a baby is fed continuously through the umbilical cord, and because their stomachs are still so small, these first weeks after being born they need to feed very often. Having the "Milk Retreat" set up can allow a mother to feed her newborn as often as possible during the day and the night. This frequent feeding and hormonal interplay coupled with keeping stress low, drinking plenty of fluids and eating lactogenic foods supports milk production.

Another way to support this early breastfeeding relationship is laid-back breastfeeding. The mother is in a semi-reclined position, propped up on pillows and blankets and the baby is placed across her. It sets them up for having good body alignment, it may make for a better latch, and gravity works with the baby.

What is the name and contact info for a highly recommended lactation consultant or IBCLC (International Board Certified Lactation Consultant)?

Who are your local breastfeeding support leaders either La Leche League or Breastfeeding USA? Leaders are available for free support by phone, text, or email (Or another free breastfeeding resource).

When and where is your local breast feeding support group meeting?

*The title "lactation consultant" is a very broad term and includes a wide range of education and skills sets, as well as models of care and commitment to breastfeeding. Your success with breast feeding may depend on this professional, so finding the right fit is important. Look for the title IBCLC and get recommendations.

breastfeeding – natural but not necessarily easy!

Feeding Your Baby

Here are some ideas to consider to support your breastfeeding or chestfeeding relationship: (you can add more ideas below)

- Spend lots of time during the first week or weeks cozied up in bed, skin-to-skin, lying down or reclining for optimal feeding positions

- Feed on demand, around the clock

- Have contact info on hand for a highly recommended lactation consultant (even if your insurance covers the hospital lactation consultant, have a back up)

- Choose health care providers that are breastfeeding-positive

- Attend a breastfeeding class during pregnancy

- Spend time around breastfeeding mothers / chestfeeding parents during pregnancy

- Attend a La Leche League or other lactation support meeting, before and after your baby is born, and have leaders contact info on hand. This is a great way to get support and wonderful way to meet other parents.

- These are helpful items to have: comfortable rocker or glider, extra pillows, body pillow, bras and shirts that can be opened easily. For leaking breasts, cloth pads and a comfy bra to hold them in place. Another option is the commercially available "Milkie Milk Savers": that fit on the breasts and collect milk that can then be frozen for later. There are many ways to dress that make breastfeeding easier, often involving layers that can either be pulled up, opened up, or pulled down.

- There are milk banks and individual mothers who make breast milk available for families that are supplementing or are not breastfeeding

- Consider avoiding pacifiers, at least until breastfeeding is established (usually 6-8 weeks), as they can interfere with latch, supply, and with learning what your baby is trying to communicate with you

- Respect your comfort level with feeding in front of others and prioritize feeding your baby over visiting with family and friends

- If you are planning on introducing a bottle, wait until breastfeeding is going well and your supply is well established (usually 6-8 weeks)

Our Stories

"When my second child was 3 months old, her poop was green, she cried a lot, and wasn't settling easily to nurse. The lactation consultant came to our home and spent an hour and a half with us. She gave us lots of helpful recommendations and followed up a couple times by email to make sure we were doing well. Later in the year, I came down with a bad case of mastitis. She made herself completely available for me to call and she guided me through to recovery without antibiotics."

all ways of feeding babies take time and devotion

Feeding Your Baby other ways

Families approach feeding their babies in many different ways and bottle feed for many different reasons. For some the choice to bottle feed is made long before their baby is born. Or this may be a choice that comes after every other effort to breastfeed has been made. Sometimes there is trauma or a mental health issues that make it unworkable. Some choose to, or end up, bottle feeding their own pumped milk. Feeding formula is another route families take. Some people buy commercial formula, or some choose to make their own at home. Donated breast milk, either through a milk bank or through community members is sometimes available. Some people use a supplemental nursing system (SNS) in order have the at the breast experience.

You may find the process of finding an alternate route is simple and straight forward or it may be a journey wrought with crisis and grief. Having the information and support needed is crucial. There are many options when it comes to types of bottles and types of nipples. A lactation consultant will have information about all feeding systems.

*There are significant health and development risks associated formula and non-human nipples.

Our Stories

"I was ready for birth to be hard, but I was completely unprepared for my breastfeeding challenges. The hospital lactation consultants tried to get the SNS to work for us, but it just felt so complicated and stressful. We ended up using formula and bottles which wasn't my first choice, but it worked for us. The hardest part was the judgement that I received and imagined from other moms.

eat like a mother!

Nourishment meals

Eating well and eating often is so important and postpartum parents often find cooking and caring for their infants and older babies (even toddlers!) quite challenging.

Who currently holds the cooking responsibilities? Meal planning, shopping, preparing, and clean up?

Who can help with these responsibilities during postpartum?

What do you love to eat or want more of in your diet?

What eating habits aren't supporting you?

eat like a mother!

Nourishment meals

After giving birth we need to be well nourished. Here are some ideas for getting support with meals. Consider all the meals: breakfasts, lunches, dinners, and snacks. Include a combination of approaches in your plan: (you can add more ideas below:

- Meal Train -meals delivered by friends and family organized by a friend using a free on-line schedule. For more information look in the appendix at the Meal Train Guide
- Frozen meals gifted at baby shower
- Freezing or canning meals yourself or with a friend
- Have lots of snacks on hand
- Family member as designated cook
- Meal delivery service
- Restaurant gift certificates
- Personal chef
- Rice cooker, crock pot, "instapot", electric kettle
- Folder of take out menus of convenient restaurants
- Basket of snacks next to the bed and a comfortable chair
- Hire a personal chef to stock the kitchen and freezer before the baby comes
- Have a set plan for breakfast foods -consider freezing frittata, quiches, and muffins

Preparing

Our Stories

"I kept a basket of snacks in bed with me for the first two weeks and after that, I had snacks at both of my "nursing stations." This helped me keep up with my body's constant demand for food!"

eat like a mother!

Nourishment meals

The foods we eat have a great impact on our immediate and long term health. When we are recovering from birth and making milk, the foods we eat affect our recovery, energy level, mental health, milk supply, and our baby's health.

Here are some ideas to consider: (you can add more ideas below)

- Drink plenty of fluids
- Eat organic foods without chemical additives
- Cooked, warm, easily digestible foods
- Variety of foods
- Plenty of "good" fats, butter, coconut oil, olive oil, etc
- Avoid or go light on caffeine, sugar, wheat, dairy, and foods you or your family are sensitive to. One sign of a food sensitivity in a baby is reflux or spit up
- Consume galactagogues, foods and beverages that promote lactation (examples: fennel and oats) and avoid foods that inhibit milk production (examples: parsley, mint, and sage)
- Look to your family or culture of origin for postpartum food traditions
- Consult with someone skilled in Chinese Medicine or Ayurveda postpartum care for dietary advice

Our Stories

"My daughter cried so much her first year. It wasn't until her one year check up that we discovered she has a dairy sensitivity. As soon as I stopped eating dairy, her temperament changed completely."

deep recovery for life long health

Health recovery

Physical recovery from pregnancy and birth involves nearly all systems of the body -muscular, skeletal, cardiovascular, endocrine, digestive, urinary, and reproductive. There are many ways we can support our bodies' natural capacity for healing.

Here are some ideas to consider: (you can add more ideas below)

- Uterine massage -massaging your belly helps your uterus return to its original size.

- Belly wrap or binding -The practice of wrapping the belly after birth to support the uterus and other organs returning to their pre-pregnancy state, as well as the abdominal muscles. One can purchase modern belly binding girdles as well as traditional wraps -or simply use a long piece of fabric, approximately 5 feet by 1 foot, wrapping and twisting every 1 and a half times around.

- Sitz baths -Warm herbal baths that the mother sits in to support the healing of the pelvic floor -tears, skid marks, hemorrhoids, etc. A midwife or herbalist can help recommend the right mix of herbs.

- Placenta encapsulation -The placenta is dried and powdered and put in capsules for the mother to take during her postpartum. Immediately after birth, a small part of the placenta can be blended with juice or a smoothie. Consumption of the placenta has anecdotally been shown to speed recovery, strengthen vitality, and balance emotions. There is concern that the placenta may have a concentration of heavy metals it has filtered during pregnancy.

- A slow return to exercise is important -listen to your body and your healthcare providers. There are physical therapists, and exercise professionals who are trained who can provide an individualized protocol. Tend to your body, and be patient with it. Consider focusing more on loving your body as it is rather than changing it.

- Staying warm and returning heat to the body -see the following page.

- Herbal pelvic steaming (vaginal or yoni steaming) is the practice of sitting over a pot of steaming herbs. The steam and volatile oils support a complete uterine cleans and healing of the organs and tissues. Finding a practitioner or looking to a family member who is carrying on the traditional practice is important because there are contradictions and sensitivities to be aware of.

For more information about recovery look to the books Natural Health after Birth by Aviva Romm and After the Baby's Birth by Robin Lim.

deep recovery for life long health

Health body work

Bodywork is a standard component of postpartum recovery throughout the world. It can help with physical recovery from birth and pregnancy, address birth-related trauma, and support mental health and over-all wellness. Get recommendations, work with practitioners that you feel really safe with, and prioritize practitioners who will come to your home.

Here are some modalities to consider: (you can add more ideas below)

- Craniosacral Therapy is a gentle, noninvasive bodywork modality that works with the craniosacral system. It can help postpartum women recover emotionally from their birth experiences, as well as supporting the return of strength, alignment, and mobility.

- Pelvic Floor Work supports recovery of the pelvic bowl. Holistic Pelvic Care addresses physical and energetic blockages in the pelvic bowl, supporting physical and emotional recovery from birth.

- Acupuncture can support overall recovery, emotional balance, and immune support

- Maya Abdominal Massage is an external non-invasive manipulation that repositions internal organs that have shifted, encouraging the flow of blood, lymph, nerve, and chi. This modality was developed by Rosita Arvigo based on her time studying with the Maya healer Don Elijio Panti. Energetic and hands-on healing of the uterus and belly can be found throughout Mexico and Central America.

- Massage can help with emotional support, muscle tension and pain, and overall relaxation

- Energy work

- Foot rubs from partner or friends

Our Stories

"I did not give myself the time to fully recover from birth. My hemorrhoid issue became so painful that it developed into anal stenosis —the closing of the anus. At 3 months postpartum I began a 5 five series Holistic Pelvic Care treatment plan from Tami Kent PT. This gentle therapy saved my butt!!"

deep recovery for life long health

Health postpartum warmth

Warming mothers after birth may be one of the oldest and most common postpartum practices found throughout the world. This includes staying in a warm environment, eating warming foods, and actively returning heat to the mother's body. It is also about avoiding cold: weather, cold food, drinks, and ice. This warmth supports recovery and long term health. Warmth may promote rest, help discharge excess fluid, reduce uterine bleeding and discharge, restore the organs to their original tone and size, and support the immune system (Natural Health after Birth by Aviva Jill Romm). American midwives have given the name "mother roasting" to these warming practices based on the Southeast Asian traditions, such as placing coals under the mother's bed or applying heat directly to her abdomen.

IMPORTANT With the more advanced techniques of adding heat, please work with either a knowledgeable family member who holds ancestral wisdom or consult with a trained practitioner.

To learn more about these concepts look to Chinese Medicine, Ayurveda, and postpartum traditions from around the world.

Here are some suggestions to consider: (you can add more ideas below)

- Dress warmly, stay inside, out of cold weather, avoiding the wind
- Use a hot water bottle on the belly and sacrum
- Drink warm drinks and food, avoiding ice and chilled foods/drinks
- Eat and drink warming types of foods such as cinnamon, ginger, and turmeric
- Have a thermos of hot tea next to the bed or nursing station
- Receive a moxabustion treatment, a Chinese Medicine practice of burning mugwart over the skin for deep heat penetration
- Warm salt rubs on abdomen
- Warm herbal baths
- Vaginal steams
- Sitz baths
- Warm oil massage
- Heating pad (don't put the baby on or near it!)
- Warm rice or salt packs

Health transitioning body

The postpartum body is in a slow return to a non-pregnant state, passing through phases of unrecognized transitions. Our changing bodies need our patience, our gratitude and our presence. While external and internalized cultural messages may be telling us otherwise, our bodies are strong and beautiful.

While a slow return to physical activity over the first year is important, too much, too soon can lead to serious health issues. Wait until six weeks to start significant exercise beyond walking and light stretching. Listen to your body. Focus on feeling presence and joy in your body, not on changing it. Find movement practices that are gentle and/or geared towards postpartum bodies. Pay particular attention and give care to your pelvic floor and your abdominal muscles. Get the support of a physical therapist or other professional who is educated in postpartum recovery. You can get a prescription for physical therapy from your doctor before leaving the hospital. Look for ways to get your needs met for movement with your baby on or near you.

Here are some movement practices to consider: (you can add more ideas below)

- Walking
- Restorative yoga
- Swimming or water exercise
- Tai chi
- Qi Gong
- Mamalates
- Belly dancing

deep recovery for life long health

Health family health

Eventually your baby will be putting everything in their mouths and the colds and flus will help build their immune system. But in this early phase sickness in the family can make everything so much more difficult. Families with older siblings, who may have exposure to a lot of viruses, are that much more vulnerable to sickness. Research natural ways to build your family's immune system with herbs and supplements, such as echinacea, black elderberry, and mushroom complex.

Write up a family sickness protocol: what do you do for colds and flus?

Here are some ideas to consider:

- All family members and visitors can wash hands upon entering the house.
- Stock up on the supplies that are part of your family's sickness protocol.
- Request sick family members and friends to keep their distance -even with just a runny nose.
- Find a healthcare provider, family member, friend, or on-line resource to have on hand for information as you need it.

What else can you do to support your overall family health?

how we feel is important

Mental Health *emotions*

The breadth and depth of emotions during postpartum is unlike any other time. Know that the huge mood swings, weepiness, strange and anxious day dreams, and complete overwhelm are normal and are all the more reason to take good care and receive lots of support. And please, do not let the idea of it all being normal stop you from reaching out for the support or professional help you need.

It is also important to know about perinatal mood and anxiety disorders (PMAD's) which include depression, anxiety, obsessive-compulsive disorder (OCD), bipolar mood disorders, and psychosis. Symptoms of PMAD's can begin during pregnancy or any time during the first year postpartum. Post traumatic stress disorder (PTSD) is a separate diagnosis which can result from a traumatic birth, separation from baby, time in the NICU, or significant breastfeeding challenges. Because traumatic stress is accumulative, previous trauma is a risk factor for postpartum PTSD. PMAD's are actually quite common at a rate that ranges from 1 out of every 5 - 8 birthing people according to Postpartum Support International (PSI). While it can feel very isolating and scary to face mental health issues with a newborn in arms, there are a lot of resources available including the PSI warmline 1.800.944.4773, local support groups, and therapists whose focus is maternal health. Therapy and medication help many mothers. Self-harm and suicidal ideation can be symptoms of various PMAD's. The National Suicide Prevention hotline is 1-800-273-8255.

What are your local resources for PMAD's and PTSD? Is there a maternal health therapist in your community? Write down names and contact info.

Who in your circles of support do you feel most comfortable talking to about your emotions? List friends, family members, and professionals.

Our Stories

"I had severe postpartum depression and had people coming to help with food and laundry. I wish I had known about postpartum depression and known that many other women have similar experiences. Perhaps all pregnant women should be told about it, so we do not end up feeling bad. Perhaps more research on postpartum depression and the causes associated with the different symptoms. I believe mine was due to low protein, and wish I would have known this."

how a mother feels is important

Mental Health emotions

When you are having a hard time, slow down and lower your stress. Be gentle with yourself and seek support. You may need to use your slow down dial, your loud speaker, and maybe even your white picket fence.

While having moments alone to reground are important, it may be more focused time with your baby that soothes your nerves. This could look like strapping your baby on and dancing, going for a walk, a warm bath together, or snuggling in bed. Know that your need for closeness with your baby is rooted in a biochemical interplay that is strengthening your bond. For some mothers separation can be more harmful than helpful.

Here are some ideas to consider. Feel free to circle the ones you like, cross out the ones you don't: (you can add more ideas below)

- See a therapist
- Give yourself permission to take medication if needed
- Find ways to get more sleep, like sleep when your baby sleeps, even in the middle of the day
- Make sure that you are eating well
- Get exercise appropriate to your recovery
- Find new mom's groups that meet up regularly
- Receive bodywork and/ or acupuncture
- Tend to your body and physical health
- Find a simple daily practice that calms you
- Choose someone to tell your birth story to with all the details and feelings
- Steer clear of negativity: avoid the news and negative conversations
- Find simple ways to treat yourself: face cleanser, pretty robe, flowers, soft sheets
- Appreciate all that your body is doing
- Set-up an "A-Team" -see glossary

Preparing

home is where the heart is

Home nesting

Every time we have a baby we re-inhabit our home in a deeper way. We naturally spend more time at home and even begin to identify more with our home. Use your nesting energy to make your home feel like what you want it to be. This is not a call for remodels or decorating make-overs. It is a reminder to make your home a safe haven for you. Identify what needs to shift for it to reflect beauty and give you a sense of peace. Make a space for your baby, and don't forget to make space for the fullness of who you are.

Where in your home feels stagnant or cold or a source of stress?

What do these places need?

Here are some ideas to consider: (you can add more ideas below)

- Switch out your chemical cleaners and personal products for natural ones.
- Minimize electromagnetic fields including Wi-Fi by using cords and/or making it easier to turn on/off.
- Clean and de-clutter, think about simplifying.
- Make sure you have 1-2 comfortable places to sit with your baby.
- Make sure you have something pleasing to look at in places you will be sitting or lying for long periods of time.

home is where the heart is

Home cleaning

Planning and communication can alleviate the stress and conflict that house cleaning can cause in a family.

Are there currently issues around cleaning? How can these be addressed?

Here are some ideas to consider: (you can add more ideas below)

- Lower your cleanliness standards (at least temporarily)
- Be clear with your partner or support people about your expectations -and that you won't be able to do your normal share of the work
- Put a to-do list on the wall for visitors to choose from
- Hire a house cleaner to come once before and after the baby comes
- Hire a house cleaner to come on a regular basis
- Get diaper service
- Have 3 friends to call when you need a little help
- Have a friend coordinate friends to do household help. This could be one person to come and do laundry the first two weeks, or people to help in the garden, or help with dishes when friends deliver meals.
- Hire a postpartum doula whose services cover household duties

each baby born changes the whole family

Family older children

The birth of a new sibling has a huge impact on a child's life. It affects the amount of time and attention parents can offer and the rhythms of family life. During pregnancy can be an optimal time for a family to ground their parenting philosophies with more practical tools. Having a new baby sibling may bring about new behavioral challenges. Small children may benefit from a low stress routine that allows for ample time for attention and play. Parents with a newborn and older children may feel stretched to their limit as they juggle everyone's needs.

Here are some ideas to consider: (you can add more ideas below)

- Create a circle of support for the older children. Set up a "kid-train" (a play date sign-up like a meal Train). Ask a family member or nanny to provide some extra care. Arrange for another family to come weekly for a full day of playing and supporting the mother-baby duo.

- Lower your child's stress. Investigate food sensitivities and allergies and consider avoiding these as well as sugar and food coloring. Resist the temptation to "make-up for" the new baby with overly exciting activities that may over stimulate the child.

- Create or continue little rituals that will refill the child's "mama cup". These can be a morning snuggle, a certain song before a meal, regular story time, or tea time. Make it dependable.

- Find ways that the older child can participate in baby care. Allow him or her to pick out the baby's clothes, massage the baby's feet, pat the baby's back.

- Watch your words and don't let the baby steal the show. While the baby's needs do become central, it is important not to make every disappointing or disciplining statement about the baby. Instead of saying "we can't go to the park because of the baby" say "Today it doesn't work to go to the park, but we will soon". Instead of "Stop making so much noise, you'll wake the baby" you can say "lets read a story right now and then you can play the drums when Papa comes home". When other people are doting on the baby, be sure to speak up about the older children, introducing them, giving them a loving touch.

- Read up on parenting books. Siblings without Rivalry by Adele Faber and Elaine Mazlish specifically addresses sibling issues and is excellent as is their other book How to Talk So Kids Will Listen & Listen So Kids Will Talk. There are so many other parenting books that may be helpful. Here are a few suggestions: Becoming the Parent You Want to Be by Laura Davis and Janis Keyser, Simplicity Parenting by Kim John Payne, Playful Parenting by Lawrence J. Cohen, Unconditional Parenting by Alfie Kohn, and Positive Discipline by Rebecca Eanes.

Our Stories

"My little guy had such a hard time not biting the baby. Finally, it was recommended that we try taking him off of wheat and that made all the difference for him. It was so stressful for all of us."

each baby born changes the whole family

Family older children

Some questions to explore are:

What currently causes your children stress?

How can these causes be lessened during postpartum?

What supports their wellbeing?

Who can help with their care?

What little rituals or rhythms are currently in practice or what would you like to create?

Our Stories

"I was so grateful to our family friend for taking our older son for so many hours, but then when he returned home he hadn't eaten lunch and was falling apart. I wish that we had communicated better and had him come home sooner."

each baby born changes the whole family

Family the grandparents

The complexity that comes with three generations can be huge.
Use this page (or on a separate sheet of paper for privacy!) to list the grandparents. Next to their names write down anything that comes to mind - how they may be most helpful, how they currently or may potentially add stress.

Here are some ideas to consider: (you can add more ideas below)

- Have clear communication about visits.
- Ask for help in specific ways.
- Find ways to express appreciation for what they are offering.
- Be strong and gentle in stating your parenting choices.

money changes everything

Money

Our financial situations change with the birth of each child. We are able to work less, or not at all, or we are paying someone else to be with our children. During the immediate postpartum and even years into the future, we may be financially dependent on our partner in a way we have never experienced. This is huge! Whatever your particular situation, it is important to address the coming financial changes. As you look at your financial priorities, consider making your wellbeing central. Maybe before you wouldn't have paid someone to come and clean for you, but now with a tiny baby, you realize that lowering your stress is worth the expense. Or maybe you are not used to paying health care providers out of pocket, but your baby is having such a hard time nursing, that it is time to call that highly recommended lactation consultant, and know that there is nothing more valuable than health and happiness.

These are conversations to have with your partner during pregnancy. Talk about a budget for postpartum support and care.

When it comes to spending there are two main forces at play: how much money we have and how much we are willing to spend. This can be teased apart.

If there actually isn't enough money to meet your postpartum goals there are creative ways to approach this.

Here are some ideas to consider: (you can add more ideas below)

- Find services for sliding scale.
- Take full advantage of your insurance. You can get a prescription for physical therapy to help with recovery. You may be able to get acupuncture and massage.
- Seek out students who may offer services for free or at a lower cost.
- Trade -many small businesses and practitioners are open to trading.
- Free clinics -ask around in your community.
- Free resources such as La Leche League and Postpartum Support International.
- Prioritize your money for support over stuff: find as much as you can second hand and hand-me-down.
- Set up a gift registry so that your family and friends can give cash instead of presents.

money changes everything

Money

Here are some ideas to consider: (you can add more ideas below)

- Sit down with your partner to discuss, plan, prioritize, and budget.
- Look at feelings and fears.
- Set aside a money for the unexpected.

How are my finances changing?

How do I feel about this?

money changes everything

Money

In preparing for a new baby, what am I spending money on? What will I be spending money on after the baby comes?

How will my spending habits change with a new baby?

How can my choices with spending support my vision of my postpartum time?

Our Stories

"I am so grateful to my husband for supporting my wellbeing. I was struggling so much after he went back to work, so we decided that instead of a family vacation the following year we would hire a postpartum doula. Her presence helped me lower my stress and be present with our daughter."

the work we do for money

Back to Work

Returning to work may present complex external factors involving finances, a position, a career or business, and the need for childcare. The internal experience may be emotional, often with conflicting feelings. For many mothers straddling work and mothering is an on going challenge and there isn't one right way to go about finding balance.

In consideration of the postpartum time, exploring your options is important. Having clarity around why you are returning may help determine what your options are. We return to work for many reasons: finances, job security, professional viability, maintaining a business, sense of identity or purpose, and even self care.

Because it is so common to need, or to want more time, it can be helpful to ask the following questions:

Why am I returning?

How long of leave is optimal for my work?

How long would I like to have?

How long would be possible?

What could be done in the case that more time is needed or wanted?

Is there any flexibility around a gradual return?

Are there ways of adjusting my financial situation or budget in order to allow for more time off?

Some work scenarios allow for creativity in making the return easier. Here are some possible strategies. You can add more ideas below)

- Bring your baby with you
- Have your baby brought to you for feeding
- Go to your baby during your lunch hour
- Arrange your schedule so that your week is broken up with a day off in the middle to be with your baby
- Slowly, over many weeks, build your hours and days to your full work load
- Go back to work at the end of the workweek so that you and your baby can ease into it
- Look for ways of working from home

the work we do for money

Back to Work

There are many ways to ease this transition. The more planning and preparing you can do while pregnant, the more you can focus on recovery and your baby during your postpartum time. It is important to talk to your boss before your baby is born about your needs for time off, creative strategies in returning, and about your pumping needs.

Here are more ideas to consider: (you can add more ideas below)

- If you will be pumping milk, begin storing up milk before you return.
- Make a plan about pumping at work and know your rights -you have the right to a private place and to breaks for pumping.
- Introduce a bottle after breastfeeding is going well.
- Nurse at night which can be made easier by sleeping with your baby.
- Offer your baby the breast a lot while you are together -more than you think they need nutritionally.
- Give your baby a chance to get to know the caregiver before you return to work.
- Clear your plate of any extra responsibilities.

Being self-employed or working at home has both advantages and disadvantages. It can be harder to feel ok about taking a maternity leave. Images of women working with babies strapped on may make you think you can, or should jump back to work right away. It is important to break down your responsibilities and determine how long you can take off for each one specifically. What can be put off? What can be delegated? This needs to be set up in advance. It may be worth the money to keep your business strong to hire someone to carry out your responsibilities. You may not be in the best condition physically, mentally, or emotionally to do what you normally do.

being prepared doesn't make it happen

The Unexpected

Planning for rest and support during the postpartum is not a guarantee that everything will go as you would like. The plan needs to be a living and responsive document, ready to adapt to the challenges that come. By setting up a circle of support beforehand, it can become easier to reach out and ask for help when you really need it. When faced with unexpected challenges, it's time to implement and call on the Postpartum Net part of the plan!

> ### *potential unexpected challenges*
> traumatic birth • cesarean birth • homebirth hospital transport • premature or sick baby
> NICU • significant feeding challenges • vaginal or pelvic floor issues • PTSD
> PMAD or perinatal mood and anxiety disorders • relationship challenges • unrelated family crisis

During pregnancy, while you are planning, consider the idea that you can work towards the birth and postpartum time that is your ideal AND prepare yourself for other outcomes. For example, if you are planning a homebirth, you could tour the hospital in the event that you do transfer, have a hospital bag packed beforehand, and even learn about your options with a non-emergency cesarean birth. Or you may set up a meeting with a recommended lactation consultant or a therapist who specializes in maternal mental health. These steps won't prevent the unwanted outcome, but they may lessen your fears, and if the unwanted outcome does happen you may find it much easier to get the help you need.

If you are faced with unexpected challenges, here are some ideas to consider:

1. Allow yourself to feel all feelings that come up. It is possible to feel grateful for being alive, love for your baby, and to feel tremendous grief, fear, anger, or despondency.
2. Use your "slow down dial". If there are any other causes of stress that can be eliminated, do. Focus on today.
3. Get all the help you can -use your "loud speaker". Don't suffer in silence. Make sure to keep your health care providers in the loop.
4. "Back to Basics" -Give you and your baby an extended in-bed period.

What is a traumatic birth? A birth is considered traumatic if the person giving birth at any time believes that their or the baby's life is in danger or if they feel emotionally or physically mistreated. The catch here is with the word "believe". This belief can be rooted in our minds or our bodies -the physiological trauma response can happen with both. Trauma is physiological, and may be compounded by psychological affects, but is not solely based in thought or emotions. The affects of trauma, referred to as post traumatic stress, are common, varied and accumulative, and can develop into post traumatic stress disorder (PTSD). The symptoms and treatment are outside of the scope of this workbook, though many of the care practices and healing modalities recommended support healing. Do seek professional mental health support.

only the essential

Back to Basics

When there has been or is currently a significant challenge "back to basics" can be a powerful tool.

This means just sleeping, eating, feeding, and being together. Get back in bed. Practice kangaroo care: spend time skin to skin; soaking each other up, all senses filled by one another. Whether you are healing from a cesarean or you and your baby went through unwanted separation, this can be a restart. It can be a very affective way to overcome feeding challenges, like latch and supply.

It may be of huge benefit to you and your baby to have a "back to basics" time even after the challenge is over. This can be a time of bonding and healing. A time to recapture your postpartum vision. Maybe it is one afternoon that you spend in bed. Or maybe it is three weeks in and near the bed. You may need two postpartum periods -one to survive and one to thrive!

This does require significant support and can be part of the Postpartum Net.

Preparing

Our Stories

"In retrospect, I realize that I didn't want to tell my midwives what a hard time I was having because I wanted them to see me as a "good mom". I didn't want them to see me as a failure. Sadly, this got in the way of them helping me."

all birth is sacred

Cesarean Recovery

A cesarean birth is major abdominal surgery, so postpartum recovery needs extra attention. It's important to follow surgery recovery protocols and allow for more time, rest, and support. The birthing parent, and therefore the baby, is in a vulnerable state and requires more care. According to WHO the cesarean rate is at one out of every three births in the United States. It makes sense for everyone to have some basic information on hand about the procedure and about the recovery. There are three types of Cesarean: planned, non-emergency, and emergency. For parents who are not planning a cesarean, it may be well worth researching ways of lowering the likelihood of having a cesarean, or if you have had one already, looking into VBAC (vaginal birth after cesarean) or HBAC (home birth after cesarean). The International Cesarean Awareness Network (ICAN) is a nonprofit that provides education, cesarean recovery support, and promotes VBAC. VBAC Facts is a non biased, research based information resource. Homebirth Cesarean (HBC) is another useful resource for recovery and support for women who planned an out of hospital birth and transferred during pregnancy or labor and had a cesarean. There is an active HBC facebook group that includes parents and professionals.

There are many ways to make a cesarean a more positive experience, prioritizing the birthing person's wellbeing and voice, as well as, bonding and breastfeeding. Hospitals have varying protocols, so it is important to talk to your provider about your preferences before hand. It is worth noting that while some of these may seem minor, they can have a big impact on how a mother later feels about her birthing experience and on her breastfeeding experience.

With a planned cesarean, families have a greater opportunity for fine tuning their vision and communicating this with the hospital staff. It makes sense for families planning a vaginal birth to learn about their options and include their cesarean preferences in their birth plans.

Here are some options to consider for before, during, and after birth. Circle or underline options that you wish to include in your birth and postpartum plans. Write in any additional ideas.

Before Surgery ~ideas to consider~
With non-emergency cesareans a mother can ask for a few minutes alone with her support people (partner, doula, etc.) To discuss any reasons for or against the decision and identify any questions about options, or lingering doubts. Take this time to come to a strong yes, or ask for more information.

Our Stories

"I wish I had known how physically intense it would be. My teeth were chattering, and afterwards I couldn't stop shaking for hours. In talking about it later, I realized that this is the only surgery of this type that is done with a person conscious. Even for surgeries much more minor, people are put under. I am glad that I asked for humane treatment and received it. People are calling this a "Gentle Cesarean" — I think "humane" is a better word!"

being prepared doesn't make it happen

Cesarean Recovery

During Surgery ~ideas to consider:

- Ask to have two support people be present. If that's not possible, the second support person can be waiting and ready to offer support as soon as the baby is born.
- Consider playing music of your choice.
- Ask that the medical staff only have conversation related to the surgery.
- Place all IV's and straps on the non-dominant arm so that the dominant arm can touch and hold the baby once born.
- Ask for medications that are approved for breastfeeding.
- As the baby is being born drop the drape or use a clear drape so that the mother can witness her baby's birth.
- Have hospital staff say when they are making the first incision, when they are going to make the incision into the uterus, and when they are lifting the baby out.
- Have the hospital staff not announce the sex of the baby.

Once Born ~ideas to consider:

- Place baby on the birth parent's chest for immediate skin-to-skin while surgery is being completed -if not possible let partner have skin-to-skin.
- Delayed cord clamping.
- Pre-birth vaginally cultured gauze to swab the baby in for microbiome transfer.
- Have all newborn tests on mother's chest if possible.
- The partner can follow and be with the baby during any procedures.
- Have the 2nd support person there to be with the mother, put their hands on her and talk to her.
- Any photography can be done by a 3rd person.
- Keep birthing person, baby, and partner together in the recovery unit to allow for bonding and breastfeeding.
- Ask for a post surgery cloth tube to help hold the baby on the mother's chest.
- If the family wants the placenta, ask that the lab take one slice and return the rest without chemicals added.

Recovery Extenders

all birth is sacred

Cesarean Recovery

The recovery period varies greatly, from one woman to the next. Go slow, be patient, and listen to your body and to your health care providers.

2-4 Days in the Hospital ~ideas to consider~
During these days a family is very much on the "flotation device." Follow the recommendations to rest, wiggle feet, raise feet, get up and walk, wear the belly wrap/binder, and take the stool softeners. In addition to the standard postpartum experiences, there may also be itchiness, swollen legs and feet, "gas pains," nausea, and pain.

Feeding can be more challenging with the incision, making a comfortable position difficult, or the baby may be lethargic and need help staying awake to nurse. Getting the baby to the breast quickly and as much as possible in the hours following birth will support breastfeeding. Ask for help. Most hospitals have a lactation consultant available to support breastfeeding and if further help is needed contact another IBCLC who comes to you highly recommended.

Returning home ~ideas to consider~
Have a "house fairy" come and tidy your house and leave a warm pot of soup on the stove, and have someone there to welcome you home. This is particularly important for a homebirth cesarean, and in this case make sure that all birth supplies have been cleared out, with no remaining signs of labor. Upon returning home, get back in bed, go "back to basics". Rest and allow for as much support as possible.

The Weeks to Follow ~ideas to consider:

- Get more help, sleep as much as you can
- Do not lift anything heavier than your baby and refrain from household work, and vigorous activity
- Rest, put feet up, walk around
- Drink lots of water, eat well, and include bone broth to help with recovery
- Continue to take the medications
- Continue to wear the belly wrap/binder
- Keep a pillow or rolled up towel near by to hold the belly for laughing, sneezing, coughing, or standing up
- Go down stairs backwards to reduce strain on abdominal muscles
- Keep the incision clean and dry
- Once the incision is healed and the scab has gone away massage the scar to help it heal more fully
- Know the warning signs of infection, such as fever, and call your provider if you have any questions
- Time a dose of pain meds so that you are not in pain when you arrive home

all birth is sacred

Cesarean Recovery

And Beyond ~ideas to consider~

Some birthing people report feeling pain from their scars for years. To support the healing of the scar consider the following:

- Self massage
- Uterine / organ massage modalities
- Acupuncture
- Holistic Pelvic Work
- Myofascial scar work

Emotions

Among people who have had cesareans there is a huge range of emotional responses. Even for one woman the complexity of her postpartum emotional landscape can be vast and unpredictable. Cesarean birth can contribute to PMAD's (perinatal mood and anxiety disorders). Some people experience PTSD (post traumatic stress Disorder) while many others have post traumatic stress symptoms.

Here are some ideas and resources that may be helpful:

- Mental health provider trained in healing trauma and or with a focus on maternal wellbeing.
- Craniosacral Therapy
- Acupuncture
- Pelvic Floor Work
- Uterine / organ massage modalities
- Massage
- Therapy
- Support group (ICAN etc.)
- Mom's groups
- See resources in the appendix

Our Stories

"I seriously over did things my first two days home, I was still taking my heavier pain meds and couldn't feel anything, so I was all over the place. I had heavy bleeding and made myself hurt worse than I would have if I had just stayed on my couch! Try to stop taking the heavier pain meds as soon as you can stand it. A little discomfort is a good reminder of the trauma your body has been through and that you need to rest!"

the synergy of the staff, the machines, and the parents

NICU the neonatal intensive care unit

Babies born before 37 weeks are considered premature. Every week of gestation is critical for development. The earlier a baby is born the higher the risks are for short term and long term challenges. Whether a baby is premature or is facing other health issues, the advanced medical science and highly specialized skill set that the NICU staff provide are nothing short of miraculous.

The development and growth of a premature baby is dependent upon the synergy of medical staff, the medical machines, and the parents. How this comes together changes as a baby grows and develops. The parenting that mothers of preemies must do looks much different than full term babies. And it is vitally important.

Even micro preemies (born before 25 weeks) can begin bonding. They need to smell their mothers (something with a birth parent's scent can be placed in the isolette), hear their birth parents, and when they are ready, be touched by their mothers. Their parents' observations are important because they are the most consistent people involved with their baby's care. These babies need their parents' advocacy and voice.

When ready, these babies benefit from their mother's milk which must be pumped until they have developed the ability to breastfeed.

When they are stabilized enough to be held, kangaroo care can begin. Kangaroo care is holding the baby skin to skin, on a parent's chest inside the shirt. The benefits are numerous and it can be done as often and long as possible.

Having a premature baby or a baby in the NICU is traumatic and exhausting, often resulting in PTSD. These birth parents' personal needs for rest, support, and healing are huge. While the hospital is providing a tremendous amount of support, it may seem too hard to ask for more, and yet these mothers and their families absolutely need more support.

When families bring their babies home from the NICU, these first weeks home can be claimed as the "milk retreat," the time for postpartum rest and bonding, a time to settle into life together.

Our Stories

"My son's case was short, and he was comparatively healthy (not a preemie), and we had tons of support, but there's still residual trauma for all of us (me, partner, sibling, kiddo) two years later. Addressing and treating the trauma that comes with having a hospitalized newborn is important."

the synergy of the staff, the machines, and the parents

NICU the neonatal intensive care unit

Here are some suggestions for considering.

- Before you see your baby have your partner or support person take a photo of the NICU and explain what is happening. This way you may experience less shock upon seeing your baby in the isolette connected to so many wires.

- Communicate with the medical staff. Keep a journal in which notes can be taken on all the information that is given to you. Ask the staff to help you understand signs that your baby is improving or when they are having a problem. Write down your questions, no matter how small, and make sure to ask them. Write down meanings of the acronyms. And speak up when you feel the need.

- Consider pushing for kangaroo care as early as possible. Research shows that it is beneficial much earlier than many hospitals' staff are comfortable with.

- You must take care of your self. Sleep as much as you can. Do your postpartum care. Eat well. Get a massage or other body work modalities that will decrease your stress and address the trauma you may be experiencing. Feel your feelings, allow for grief and fear. Keep a personal journal to help process your emotional experience.

- You won't be able to be there with your baby all the time. Taking the time away to take care of yourself is crucial.

- You can ask to be present during tests and you can make a point of being present when the nurses make their rounds.

- Take full advantage of everything being offered -any meals, showers, lactation support, occupational therapy, and the social worker on staff.

- Breastfeeding even if your baby is able to, may be challenging. It may be harder than expected. Pumping is a lot of work and building your supply may prove to be hard. Continue to get help from a lactation consultant and follow supply building protocols.

- Get the support of a family member or postpartum doula to help you manage everything.

- Tune out all the beeping.

- Put someone else in charge of keeping people updated -your "postpartum PR" either through group emails, a facebook page, or a blog.

- Connect with other NICU parents on-line or in person.

- Find a rhythm for caring for and connecting with your older children

- Use the BRAIN tool: Benefits, Risks, Alternatives, and doing Nothing.

- Trust your instincts

Our Stories

"The complexity of how I felt was immense: happiness at having just given birth and also extreme sadness and distress at having a long NICU stay with my micro-preemie."

with more babies, you need more hands

Multiples

With twins or triplets the need for setting up postpartum support ahead of time is crucial. Fill your circles with professionals and friends who understand multiples. And remember that self care is essential and requires support.

Plan on ONLY being responsible for feeding, eating, and sleeping. If you are breastfeeding, know that you must eat a tremendous amount of food. For at least the first two weeks at home arrange to have someone there with you around the clock. This could be a schedule of friends and family members, or someone from out-of-town staying with you, or a postpartum doula. Having live-in support is ideal. You will need help during the night. If possible, ease off the support gradually.

Here are some suggestions to consider before the babies come: (you can add more ideas below)

- Research: -read books, blogs, connect with other multiple moms in person and on line.
- Meet with an IBCLC who is knowledgeable about multiples.
- Find local multiples groups to connect with. They will have hand-me-downs, advice, and other support.
- Find multiples groups on-line.
- Cesarean birth and the NICU are common, so it is especially important to learn about these before hand and make plans accordingly.
- Baby gear that some mothers recommend: "My Best Friend Twins Nursing Pillow", "Twin Z Pillow", swings, boppy pillow-nests, snap+go stroller, and car seat canopies.
- Tour the hospital, including the NICU even if you are planning a homebirth, and meet with the social worker to discuss options and resources.

Our Stories

"You just have to accept that parenting multiples is different. I longed to just hold one baby and totally soak her up —but I had to keep moving, on to the next. In order to keep them fed I had to pump —but I really just wanted to hold them and not be hooked up to the pump. You do what you have to do."

with more babies, you need more hands

Multiples

Here some suggestions to consider for after the babies come: (you can add more ideas below)

- If breastfeeding is a goal use your time in the hospital, with all the extra support to establish breastfeeding and practice tandem nursing.

- If one baby can go home and one has to stay in the NICU, plan for separate postpartum times for each baby's arrival home with support, time to bond, and adjust.

- If staggered discharge is necessary, use technology to stay connected and when each baby comes home allow for a set time adjusting or bonding, consider baby mooning and extend your "milk retreat".

- Once home consider doing "back to basics". This can be done if there has been a rough beginning for breastfeeding or any kind of separation. Once a baby is effectively breastfeeding take the baby to bed for several days of around the clock feeding. Breastfeed the other babies a few times a day and then go back to your normal feeding pattern and rotate in another baby when you are ready to do another round of "baby mooning".

- Work at putting babies on the same feeding and sleep schedules. While at the hospital have them bring all the babies to each feeding when possible. Later on if one wakes in the middle of the night, wake the others to feed.

- Setup multiple baby-stations throughout the house so that you don't have to leave one baby to get a diaper.

- Co-bedding (babies sleep together) when physically stable: this supports babies in regulating body systems and syncing their sleep/wake cycles. Or put their cribs or incubators together to make parenting them easier.

- Put babies names on their incubators or cribs and get to know each baby's reactions and behaviors and encourage the staff to as well.

- Make a household help to-do list, print out many copies, and each day put up a new one for your help.

- If you are pumping, use the hospital grade pump. Set up a pumping station in the house and have a kit in the car.

- Have a crate in the car with the baby gear: clothes, diapers, blankets.

- Remember bonding happens over a long time. Know that less responsive babies may need extra focus.

The Plan *putting it all together*

The plan weaves together all aspects of your life and the people in it. It is based on what you know now about the weeks to come after your baby is born. It is flexible and strong, ready to adapt to the challenges that arise.

The first two plan template sheets are the Milk Retreat and the Postpartum Net. You can work with this in whatever way feels best to you. Maybe you use these to jot down ideas as you're working through the workbook, or maybe you condense the following template pages into a succinct two page plan. Remember, the Milk Retreat is essentially *how you want it to go* and the *postpartum net* is there to help you through whatever challenges arise.

As you determine who is helping with what, make sure to ask them ahead of time. Get your inner circle of support on board with your plan, or if need be, plan around their lack of support. While you deserve to be supported, some people may not be available in the ways you would like. This can be frustrating, but ultimately it is gratitude for the support we do have that keeps us strong.

Get specific with your time lines and your tasks.

Know who you will contact when things get hard.

Having a plan doesn't guarantee an easy time, but it does set us up for the best possible postpartum time.

Claim this precious time and fill it with love.

In the space below write out the word or phrase that is your compass from the exercise on page 12.

My Compass / My Vision

Milk Retreat

A set amount of time for rest, support, and care.

Postpartum Net

Resources and plans for unexpected challenges

mental~emotional~whole body

feeding

pelvic healing

practical

Your People

General Help
close support people

postpartum doula

"postpartum PR"

Food
Meal Train Coordinator / cook / friend to call for help

Breastfeeding
free breastfeeding resources (as in La Leche League)

experienced friend

recommended IBCLC

Health + Wellbeing
midwife / primary provider

acupuncturist / body workers

3 friends or family to call when you are struggling and need to talk

mamas support group

1 close friend to tell your complete birth story

mental health resources for PMAD's: group, hotline, counselor

placenta

Home
family member or friend to call for help

professional

Childcare for older children
friend / family member / nanny / "kid-Train" organizer

Your People
Your close support people

This may be your own mother visiting for 2 weeks, your mother-in-law who lives nearby, your sister, a postpartum doula, or a friend who you hire for additional support. You may have a robust inner circle, or you may feel like you are on an island, or maybe you feel smothered by help you don't want! The point here is to reflect on your feelings and your needs, and then work out the details with each person involved.

List each person who is in this inner circle of close support and next to their name, put how long they will be supporting you (or how often) and then list out how you want to be supported by them. Maybe your mother-in-law hates to cook and has a hard time with your older children. Could she be in charge of laundry and reading to the older children? These will all need to be communicated ahead of time and possibly communicated again during. Add time lines to the calendar.

NAME	DURATION	SUPPORT TYPE

The Plan
Rest - The Milk Retreat

How long will you stay in bed or on the couch?

How long will you stay home?

How long do you plan to have off from your normal activities? (you can add these time lines to the calendar)

- paid work (if you are self employed take a separate sheet of paper and detail out your various roles)

- house work: cleaning, cooking, shopping, gardening, animal care, paying bills

- social life

- screen time / use of phone

- other interests and responsibilities (make a list)

The Plan

Food

What kind of support with meals are you planning? How are you stocking up? How long are you planning for? What foods are you planning on eating and what are you avoiding?

Health + Wellbeing

recovery care practices and modalities

avoiding cold - staying warm - adding heat

The Plan

Family

Grandparents: How will they help and what boundaries would you like to have?

Older children: Who will help you care for them? How will you ease this transition for them?

Visitor protocol

How will you stay connected? How will you draw boundaries?

The Plan

Home

What home-related responsibilities are your partner or other support people taking on?

Work

How will you prepare to go back to work?

What kind of support is needed for the transition back to work?

What are your baby care and feeding plans?

Contingency

In the case that unexpected challenges arise, how can you add more support and more rest to your plan?

The Plan
Extended Recovery:

Preferences and priorities for postpartum with a cesarean birth:
(Add your immediate postpartum and birth preferences to your birth plan)

Preferences and priorities for time in the NICU:

Multiples Addendum

Names of family, friends, and professionals who will help you for the first month and beyond. Who will be with you?

Names of professionals knowledgable about multiples: lactation consultant, postpartum doula, pediatrician.

Names of other multiple families who will be available to get support, information, and resources.

Budget

This is for non-material support: lactation consultant, housecleaning, doulas, acupuncture / Chinese Medicine, Craniosacral Therapy, pelvic floor therapies, massage, diaper service . . . etc. It is worth checking with your insurance to see what may be covered.

Must Have What are the services or care that you must have?

Total:

Contingency What are the services or care that you will need if specific challenges arise?

Total:

Sub Total:

Ideally In an ideal world what else would you want?

Total:

Grand Total:

The Plan

Calendar

Week 1

M	T	W	Th	F	S	S

Week 2

M	T	W	Th	F	S	S

Calendar

Week 3

M	T	W	Th	F	S	S

Week 4

M	T	W	Th	F	S	S

Calendar

Week 5

M	T	W	Th	F	S	S

Week 6

M	T	W	Th	F	S	S

Calendar

Week 7

M	T	W	Th	F	S	S

Week 8

M	T	W	Th	F	S	S

Calendar

Week 9

M	T	W	Th	F	S	S

Week 10

M	T	W	Th	F	S	S

Pregnancy To-Do list

too late for planning!

HELP if your baby is here!

While this workbook is designed to be worked through during pregnancy, some of you won't have it in hand until after your baby has been born.

If this is the case, use the following questions to assess where you are and what you are needing. Consider asking one of your main support people (your partner, sister, friend, postpartum doula etc.) to help you prioritize and think clearly about your circles of support and what resources you may be needing.

Identify your challenges: What is hard?

What are your immediate needs?

Who can help you?

birth is a rite of passage

Birth Considerations

While the focus of this workbook is not on the birth or immediate postpartum, it is important to be educated about your options and clear about your preferences.

Here are some topics to consider:

- Pain medication, comfort measures
- Cesarean birth preferences
- NICU preferences
- Microbiome preferences
- Immediate skin-to-skin
- Cord clamping, placenta
- Bathing and dressing baby
- Feeding, breastfeeding, pacifiers
- Procedures and tests for the baby: determine which ones you want right away, which you will delay for an hour, which you will delay or avoid.
- Rooming in, privacy, guests

Resources

On-line

Postpartum Support International is dedicated to helping women suffering from perinatal mood and anxiety disorders, including postpartum depression, the most common complication of childbirth. They offer free support and resources: psioffice@postpartum.net or 1-800-944-4PPD.

The Fourth Trimester Project beautiful resources with everything postpartum. https://the4thtrimesterv2.squarespace.com

Global Health Media has beautiful education lactation videos. https://globalhealthmedia.org/videos/breastfeeding

La Leche League International is a wonderful site in a many languages. La Leche League offers free breastfeeding information and support through monthly meetings and on call support.

KellyMom.com informative site on evidenced based breastfeeding and parenting.

Mothering.com pregnancy, babies, natural family living and more.

M2Mpostpartum.org perserving multicultural postpartum wisdom

ICAN (International Cesarean Awareness Network) is a nonprofit organization whose mission is to improve maternal-child health by preventing unnecessary cesareans through education, providing support for cesarean recovery, and promoting Vaginal Birth After Cesarean (VBAC).

Homebirth Cesarean provides support and awareness around planned out-of-hospital births that end in cesareans, referred to as Homebirth Cesareans (HBCs).

TakeThemaMeal.com is a meal delivery organizing site because it does not require participants to create their own account.

Books

Birth
Birthing From Within by Pam England
Pregnancy, Birth and the Newborn by Simkin Whalley, and Keppler
A Thinking Woman's Guide to a Better Birth by Henci Goer
Gentle Birth, Gentle Mothering by Sarah Buckley.

Postpartum - Newborns
Mothering the New Mother by Sally Placksin
Natural Health After Birth by Avivia Jill Romm
After the Baby's Birth by Robin Lim
Lockdown by Guang Ming
The First Forty Days, by Heng Ou
Fourth Trimester by Kimberly Johnson

Breastfeeding
The Womanly Art of Breastfeeding from La Leche League
Mother Food by Hilary Jacobson
Breastfeeding Grief by Hilary Jacobson

Cesarean
Homebirth Cesarean by Courtney Jarecki
My Cesarean edited by Rachel Mortiz

Multiples
Mothering Multiples by Karen Kerkhoff Gromada

Health
Smart Medicine for a Healthier Child by Janet Zand

Mental Health
The Mother-to-Mother Postpartum Depession Support Book by Sandra Poulin
Waking the Tiger by Peter A. Levine
The Body Keeps the Score by Bessel van der Kolk

Parenting
Siblings without Rivalry and How to Talk So Kids Will Listen & Listen So Kids Will Talk by Adele Faber and Elaine Mazlish
Becoming the Parent You Want to Be by Laura Davis and Janis Keyser
Simplicity Parenting by Kim John Payne
Playful Parenting by Lawrence J. Cohen
Unconditional Parenting by Alfie Kohn
Positive Discipline by Rebecca Eanes.

Black Resources for Black, African, African American, African Diaspara

On-line

Virtual Services and Classes:
Erica Davis -childbirth ecuation, postpartum preparation classes,
https://www.wholebodypregnancy.com

Her Holistic Path -childbirth education and virtual doula: IG@herholisticpath, www.herholistcpath.com

Tassie Teaches, Unassisted Childbirth Educator: IG@tassieteaches, www.tassieteaches.wixsite.com

The Black Doula, Sabia C. Wade offers virtual full specturum doula support: www.theblackdoula.com

Black Women Do Breastfeed, support and resources: IG@bwdbf, www.blackwomendobreastfeed.org

Melissa Danielle, offers virtual full spectrum doula support, health coach: www.doulainparadise.info

Sabrina Elizabeth, Postpartum Planning Program: IG@Sabrina.womb, www.sabrinaelizabeth.info

Directories:
National Black Doulas Association a directory of doulas and other practitioners: www.blackdoulas.org

National Association of Professional and Peer Lactation Supporters of Color directory: www.napplsc.org

Sista Midwife Productions, Black midwife and doula directory: www.sistamidwife.com

Irth App, Birth With Out Bias: www.birthwithoutbias.com

Steamy Chick Directory - certified vaginal steam practitioners: www.steamychick.com/practitioners

Information:
From Mothers to Mothers ~ perserving multicultural postpartum wisdom: www.m2mpostpartum.org

Blogs:
Black Moms Blog: www.blackmomsblog.com

Care package subscriptions:
Postpartum Queen postpartum care kits: www.postpartumqueen.com
Cater to Mom, Postpartum Subscription Box + Online Community: www.catertomom.com

Books

The Mini Mocha Manual to pregnancy & Childbirth, the essential guide for Black Women by Kimberly Seals Allers.

The Mocha Manual to a Fabulous Pregnancy (plus DVD) by Kimberly Seals Allers.

Mama's Little Baby: The Black Woman's Guide to Pregnancy Childbirth, and Baby's First Year by Dennis Brown and Pamela A. Toussaint

Black, Pregnancy and loving it: The Comprehensive Pregnancy Guide, for Today's Woman of Color by Yvette Allen-Campbell and Dr. Suzanne Greenidge-Hewitt

Having Your Baby: For the Special Needs of a Black Mother-to-be, from conception to Newborn Care by Hilda Hutcherson

---

This list of resources will be maintained at: www.buildyournestworkbook.com
Please be in touch with suggestions and do share freely with no credit given.

LGBTQ Resources

On-line

Virtual Services and Classes:
Erica Davis -childbirth ecuation, postpartum preparation classes,
https://www.wholebodypregnancy.com

MAIA Midwifery: offering fertility education, consults and support groups on line. www.maiamidwifery.com

Woven Bodies: inclusive digital practice supporting queer folks and allies from family planning through parenthood: www.wovenbodies.com

Childbirth Ed on-line series / private sessions via video chat: www.birthingbeyondthebinary.com

BirthRoot on-line Childbirth Class: www.classroom.sandralondino.com

Love Over Fear Wellness: support and education, including the "Queering the Childbearing Year -A Virtual 6-Week Support Group": www.loveoverfearwellness.com

The Black Doula, Sabia C. Wade offers virtual full specturum doula support: www.theblackdoula.com

Information:
National LGBT Health Education Center: www.www.lgbthealtheducation.org/wp-content/uploads/Pathways-to-Parenthood-for-LGBT-People.pdf

Health Resources for pregnant trans people: www.seriousplayfilms.com

La Leche League: www.llli.org/breastfeeding-info/transgender-non-binary-parents

Blogs:
www.circleofmoms.com/top25/LGBT-parent

Podcasts:
www.masculinebirthritual.com

facebook groups:
The Other Box
Birthing and Breast or Chestfeeding Trans people and allies

Books

The Essential Guide to Lesbian Conception Pregnancy, and Birth by Stephanie Brill
Queer + Pregnant, a personal journal by Mx. Jenna M Brown
Lunasea Scout Guide for Breastfeeding Families by Kait Moon
The ultimate Guide to Pregnancy for Lesbians by Rachel Pepper
And baby makes more by Susan Goldberg
Confessions fo the Other Mother by Harlyn Aizley
Buying Dad: One Woman's Search for the Perfect Sperm Donor by Harlyn Aizley
Journey to same sex parenthood by Eric Rosswood
The Ultimate Guide for Gay Dads by Eric Rosswood
Subversive Motherhood by Maria Llopis
Pregnant Butch: Nine Long Months Spent in Drag by A. K. Summers
Where's the Mother: Stories from a Transgender Dad by Trevor MacDonald
Pride and Joy: a Guide for Lesbian, Gay, Bisexual, and Trans Parents by Sarah and Rachel Hagger-Holt

This list of resources will be maintained at: www.buildyournestworkbook.com
Please be in touch with suggestions and do share freely with no credit given.

A–Z

Glossary of Postpartum Terms

wellness for the mother-baby duo

The following terms are a mix of resources, healing modalities, traditional practices, aspects of postpartum and a few of my own postpartum inventions, which are in quotations. With the term "mother-baby duo" I am recognizing the interdependence and the inseparability of a birthing person and a baby's wellness.

By including traditional practices, my intention is to show that prioritizing rest, support, and care during the postpartum is found throughout the world, including in the US where many people follow their traditions. People whose families have lost their postpartum traditions can look to the wisdom of traditional practices with respect, without appropriating.

This document continues to grow and evolve. Do send me new terms to add or input on my definitions. How the postpartum is approached is deeply cultural and with my work I am hoping to nurture a culture in which we are honored and cared for after giving birth.

This glossary is available for free on my website. And finally, the content in this document is not intended to be a substitute for medical advice, diagnosis, or treatment.

"A-team" Two to four friends who have agreed to be your allies, aunties, and advocates. This is a way of bringing intentionality to friendship so that the friends can work together in providing support.

afartanbah The Somali tradition of giving mothers 40 days of nourishing food, warmth, rest, and special care in order to fully recover from birth.

afterpains Contractions of the uterus during the first week postpartum, often more painful with subsequent babies and during breastfeeding.

attachment parenting This term, coined by William and Martha Sears, is based on Attachment Theory which has come from 60 years of developmental psychology research showing a biological imperative for the mother-baby bond. Attachment parenting philosophy focuses on the nurturing connection between parents and their children. It is popularized by parenting practices that are the norm throughout the world and through out human history. These include: breastfeeding on demand, skin-to-skin, babies sleeping with or near their mother, and baby wearing.

baby wearing The practice of carrying a baby in a carrier, including fabric wraps, slings, and packs, etc. It enables a mother or other caregiver to hold the baby close, with less physical strain, and have hands free for tending to other things. Research shows that facing in is preferable for a young baby's hips and back.

belly wrapping or binding The cross-cultural practice of wrapping the mother's belly after birth. The wrapping supports the uterus and other organs and abdominal muscles in their return to a pre-pregnancy state. Other benefits may include decreased bleeding, warming of the abdomen and uterus, reduced swelling, reorienting core muscles and improved posture. Modern belly binding girdles and traditional cloth wraps are available for purchase. Or a long piece of fabric, approximately 5 feet by 1 foot, can be used by wrapping and twisting every one and a half times around.

birth doula A trained labor coach who assists mothers during labor and birth. She provides continuous emotional support, as well as assistance with other non-medical aspects of care, and can help navigate the medical choices that may arise. (See also full spectrum doula and postpartum doula)

bonding An emotional and biochemical interplay between parents, as well as other caregivers, and baby that begins immediately after birth and continues to develop over time. It builds a secure attachment for the infant supporting optimal neurological development. For parents it sets into play a hormonal chain reaction that supports responsive and loving parenting and overall maternal wellbeing.

breastfeeding grief The feelings of sadness and loss that people who plan to exclusively breastfeed feel when it doesn't happen, coined by author Hilary Jacobson.

circumcision is the surgical removal of the foreskin, the tissue covering the penis. There are many reasons parents choose not to circumcise their sons, including complications with the surgery, anesthesia, and lifelong damage to the functionality of the penis. The foreskin is a man's most erogenous zone and it also acts to protect the penis. No major medical association, including the American Medical Association, recommends it for infants, and at this point the circumcision rate in the US is at 32%.

colostrum The milky substance produced by the breasts for the first 2-4 days after birth, before true milk "comes in." It is rich with proteins, carbohydrates, fats, vitamins, minerals, proteins, as well as antibodies that protect against bacteria and viruses.

cosleeping The practice of babies and children sleeping with their parents in bed, or adjacent to the bed in a "co-sleeper". Many mothers choose to cosleep because it enables them to get more sleep, maintain their breast milk supply, and is another way to deepen their bond. There are safety practices to be aware of, including types of bedding and not exposing babies to adults who have smoked or have consumed alcohol or drugs. Sleeping with an infant on couches and in reclining chairs is not safe.

Craniosacral Therapy (CST) A gentle, noninvasive bodywork modality that works with the craniosacral system. It can help postpartum people recover emotionally from their birth experiences, as well as supporting the return of strength, alignment, and mobility to the body. For babies, a CST session can minimize or eliminate the repercussions of difficult births, addressing many health challenges that may arise including difficulty with breastfeeding.

cuarentena The Latin American tradition of giving mothers 40 days of nourishing food, warmth, rest, and special care in order to fully recover from birth.

family-centered cesarean Practices that address the emotional and physical needs of mothers and babies, specifically emotional support, bonding, breastfeeding, and microbiome transfer.

feeding on demand Following the mother's instincts and the baby's hunger cues; not feeding at set time increments. Newborns have very small stomachs and need to feed very frequently to meet their nutritional needs.

food restrictions Foods that are avoided during the postpartum either for the mother's health or for the baby's. Specific foods vary greatly culture to culture. Some commonly avoided foods are cabbage and other brassica family vegetables, caffeine, sour foods, and cold foods.

From Mothers to Mothers An organization perserving multi-cultural postpartum wisdom www.m2mpostpartum.org

full spectrum doula A doula who provides support to families through all pregnancy experiences, including birth, abortion, adoption, surrogacy, miscarriage, and stillbirth.

herbal peri-bottle A plastic squeeze bottle filled with warm sitz bath herbs, used to rinse instead of wiping with toilet paper in order to decrease irritation and support healing the injured tissues.

hind milk, fore milk The first milk that a baby gets at the beginning of a feeding is called the fore milk. As a feeding progresses the hind milk is produced with its higher fat content.

Holistic Pelvic Care™ Physical and energetic healing in the pelvic bowl, supporting physical and emotional recovery from birth. Resolving symptoms such as pelvic pain, discomfort, incontinence, hemorrhoids, or muscle weakness, and greatly assists overall healing. Pioneered by Portland-based women's health physical therapist Tami Kent. See "pelvic floor work".

homebirth cesarean A birth that was planned as an out of hospital birth and ends in cesarean.

Homebirth Cesarean An organization that provides support and awareness around planned out-of-hospital births that end in cesareans, referred to as Homebirth Cesareans (HBC). Resources include workshops for healthcare providers and mothers, an active facebook group, and book and workbook: Homebirth Cesarean and Healing from a Homebirth Cesarean.

"house fairy" A close friend, relative, or postpartum doula who is on call and ready to prepare your home for you and your newborn when you come home after the birth.

ICAN "The International Cesarean Awareness Network, Inc. (ICAN) is a nonprofit organization whose mission is to improve maternal-child health by preventing unnecessary cesareans through education, providing support for cesarean recovery, and promoting Vaginal Birth After Cesarean (VBAC)."

infant massage Nurturing touch by a parent, often including rubbing in oil, and working through the joints, and stretching the limbs. It supports bonding, development, and health. Infant massage classes taught in the US are rooted in the Indian tradition.

intrusive thoughts Strange and often disturbing dreams, images, and thoughts that mothers experience during postpartum. If relatively mild these thoughts can be part of healthy postpartum experience. If they become too frequent or strong, they may be a symptom of a Postpartum Mood and Anxiety disorder.

kangaroo care The practice of holding a baby against the chest, skin-to-skin, inside of the parent's shirt. This is especially beneficial for premature or sick babies.

La Leche League (LLL) An international nonprofit organization that offers through peer support, encouragement, information, and education. LLL promotes a better understanding of breastfeeding as an important element in the healthy development of the baby and mother.

lactation consultant A health professional who provides breastfeeding support. This is not a standardized profession and there is wide variability in level of education and type of philosophy. International Board Certified Lactation Consultants (IBCLC) go through a rigorous training and certification process.

lochia The bloody discharge lasting for 4-6 weeks postpartum. The first week is much like menstruation and then lightens as the weeks progress.

lying-in A traditional European and European American practice that gives women (often 6 weeks of) nourishing food, warmth, rest, and special care in order to fully recover from birth.

"mama-sitter" A friend, family member, or postpartum doula who comes to simply be with the mother and her new baby.

meal train An online schedule for friends and family members who have signed up to deliver meals. This can be catered to a family's diet and needs.

microbiome (human) The ecological community of microorganisms that are intrinsic to the human body. A growing body of research is showing that much of human health and wellbeing may be affected by microorganisms of the gut, with a strong correlation between greater diversity and greater health.

microbiome transfer The transfer of the birthing person's microbiome to their baby during and after birth through exposure through the birth canal, skin-to-skin contact, and breastfeeding.

"milk retreat" This is a set amount of time to receive rest, support, and care in order to fully recover from birth. It is a time to devote to feeding the baby -thus "milk retreat," and requires planning.

mother roasting Refers to specific warming practices such as moxibustion treatments and warm salt rubs. It was coined by an American midwife referring to the Southeast Asian practices of using coals and fires to warm new mothers after birth. See postpartum warmth.

moxibustion treatment A Chinese Medicine practice of burning mugwort over the skin for deep heat penetration and to activate acupuncture points. It is used during postpartum to return heat to the womb, which supports recovery and long term vitality.

nam lua in The Vietnamese postpartum tradition of laying in a bed over hot coals, and giving women nourishing food, warmth, rest, and special care in order to fully recover from birth.

"newborn map" This is the geography of your first weeks after birth, the places you feel most unguarded and truly safe. This can be the rooms of your home, the homes of family or friends, offices you visit for appointments, or public places that you love.

nursing station A bed, a comfortable chair, or couch with water, snacks, a book to read. If there are siblings, a special toy or book that come out only during feeding can be included.

pelvic floor physical therapy A branch of physical therapy that address the pelvic floor muscles through direct manipulation and excises. See holistic pelvic work.

perinatal counselor / maternal health therapist A therapist trained in addressing mental health issues that arise during pregnancy and postpartum.

Perinatal Mood and Anxiety Disorders Mental health issues that begin during pregnancy or up to two years postpartum, including depression, anxiety, OCD, bipolar mood disorder, and postpartum psychosis.

Physiologic Postpartum Care "A system of care that both follows and honors the physiologic design of postpartum women. The 'optimal results' for postpartum care is not just the survival of Mothers, but the thriving of Mothers. Physiologic Postpartum Care recognizes Mothers as the foundation of humanity, and supports Mothers life-long health and vitality in the name of continuity of Life." This term was coined by Rachelle Garcia Seliga.

placenta encapsulation/consumption The placenta is dried and powdered and put in capsules for the mother to take during her postpartum. Immediately after birth, a small part of the placenta can be blended with juice or in a smoothie. Consumption of the placenta has anecdotally been shown to speed recovery, strengthen vitality, and balance emotions.

plan C Is a term that evolved from the Homebirth Cesarean community, specifically referring to the potential of a homebirth transfer to cesarean birth, Plan C is a tool and planning guide used to address the possibility of a cesarean and identify a family's highest needs and priorities in a surgical birth. Learn more about this in the book "Homebirth Cesarean" by Courtney Jarecki.

post traumatic growth The idea that positive change is experienced as a result of the struggle with a major life crisis or a traumatic event.

"postpartum buddy" This is a friend who agrees to have regular check in's or who will join you for outings. This could be a walking partner, or a buddy to go to the breastfeeding meet-up.

postpartum depression The most common complication in childbirth, postpartum depression is a temporary and treatable depression.

postpartum doula A trained professional who provides support and guidance to a new mother and her family. This may include informational guidance and support in breastfeeding and newborn care, light household chores, meal preparation, errands, and care of mother and baby. A postpartum doula's care is catered to the family's needs.

postpartum net The contingency part of the postpartum plan that details resources for unexpected challenges and plans for extending the time of rest and support.

"postpartum pause" The moment when a postpartum mother feels ready to take on more household or work responsibilities and instead of jumping back in, she pauses to savor her newborn, her family, and this special time.

postpartum plan 1) A detailed outline of how a family will have the rest, support, and care they need and resources to help them through unexpected challenges. "Milk Retreat + Postpartum Net" 2) A section of the birth plan that outlines the choices a family has made for the care of mother and baby immediately

Postpartum Post Traumatic Stress Disorder (PTSD) Most often this illness is caused by a real or perceived trauma during delivery or postpartum and symptoms include disturbing thoughts or feelings related to past traumas. Symptoms may include intrusive re-experiencing of a past traumatic event, flashbacks or nightmares, avoidance of stimuli associated with the event, persistent increased arousal (irritability, difficulty sleeping, hyper vigilance, exaggerated startle response), anxiety and panic attacks and feeling a sense of unreality and detachment. A person can have post traumatic stress without enough symptoms to be diagnosed with PTSD.

"postpartum PR" How a family and their community publicly shares about the birth, the baby, and how the family is doing, including social media, the sharing of images, and face-to-face communication. With intentionality, privacy can be maintained and connection nurtured.

postpartum warmth The cross-cultural traditional practice that includes keeping warm, actively returning heat to the body, and avoiding cold.

proper latch Occurs when breastfeeding is effectively getting milk to the baby and is comfortable for the mother. Ongoing pain in the nipples during breastfeeding is a sign of poor latch which can result in lowering a mother's supply. There are many possible causes of a poor latch, including the use of pacifiers and artificial nipples, as well as lip and tongue ties.

P.S.I (Postpartum Support International) An organization dedicated to helping women suffering from perinatal mood and anxiety disorders including: depression, anxiety, post traumatic stress syndrome, OCD, bipolar mood disorder, and postpartum psychosis. Group chats with experts, local volunteers, support for partners, and lots of useful information on the website.

"Sibling Train" An online schedule of friends and family members who have signed up to have special time with the older siblings of a newborn.

sitz bath A warm herbal bath that supports the healing of the pelvic floor (tears, skid marks, hemorrhoids, etc). A midwife or herbalist can prescribe the right mix of herbs to address specific conditions.

skin-to-skin The practice of putting a baby directly on the parent's chest without any blankets or clothes between them. This supports the stabilization of the baby's temperature, heart rate, breathing, and blood sugar. It also supports the transfer of beneficial bacteria, seeding the microbiome. It is soothing for the parent and the baby, supports breastfeeding, milk supply, and the bonding process.

supplementing The practice of giving a breastfed baby either formula or other human breast milk. Supplementing, even a little may diminish milk production. If supplementing is needed there are often resources for securing donated milk either privately or through a free milk bank.

supply The amount of milk produced. Oversupply and undersupply are both challenges that affect mother and baby's health and wellbeing. Signs of undersupply have to do with a baby's growth as well as the number of wet and soiled diapers depending on age. Oversupply can result in engorgement and mastitis. Many things can affect supply including foods, stress, contact with baby, frequency of feeding, and type of latch.

ties This includes tongue-ties, lip-ties, and cheek-ties all of which can result in a poor latch and super painful nipples. If a tie is identified or suspected and there are breastfeeding challenges, finding a knowledgeable and supportive health care provider is important. It is worth mentioning that within the medical professions there is not a universal system of diagnosis. Two significant signs are a painful latch and lack milk transfer which is diagnosed by weighing the baby before and after a feeding.

uterine massage Massaging the belly helps the uterus return to its original size, expelling extra fluids. It is done by health care providers directly after birth and it can be continued for the following weeks by the mother.

uterine / organ massage modalities An external non-invasive manipulation that repositions internal organs that have shifted, encouraging the flow of blood, lymph, nerve and chi. There are specific modalities within in traditional Chinese and Meso-American medicine systems.

zuo yue zi Or "sitting the month" is the traditional Chinese practice of giving mothers 30 days of nourishing food, warmth, rest, and special care in order to fully recover from birth.

Meal Train Guide

Sharing food is giving love!

A Meal Train is a sign up schedule for friends and family to bring meals to the family of a newborn. It is a way for a community to participate in this special time while providing practical support.

This guide is included in my Build Your Nest postpartum planning workbook and also is available for free on my website. If you have downloaded it, I recommend printing it so that you can mark it up with your own ideas, circles and stars.

The guide gives you 3 steps:

1. *meet with the parents*: figure out what the family needs and wants

2. *create the circle*: get their friends and family on board

3. *activate and keep it coming*: get the schedule filled up and be a liaison

This same format can also be used to organize play times for older siblings -another great way to support the family of a newborn.

Please do not plan your own Meal Train!

The family of a newborn absolutely deserves to be cared for in this way. Coordinating the Meal Train is a gift to be given to a family. The role of the coordinator is to be a liaison for the family and their community. It is so much easier for a friend to say "these guys need more food, bring it on".

Something to keep in mind as you are setting up a Meal Train is that each family has a unique circle of friends and family that surround them. Some communities are familiar with Meal Trains and will quickly fill up the sign up sheet. Other communities may be unfamiliar with the Meal Train and also unaware of the needs of families with newborns. The job of the coordinator is to be creative and responsive to the specific community at hand. There are many ways to go about setting up a successful Meal Train.

*I have written this with families of newborns in mind, but Meal Trains are also very helpful for people recovering from surgery or injury, healing from a major illness, or facing the loss of a loved one. It is a powerful way of supporting friends through life's many transitions.

Meal Train Guide

Step 1: meet with the parents

Be ready to take notes because from this you will write up the "cook's instructions," which will be put in the notes on the website and can be emailed to people as well.

Before you begin gathering information from your friend, take a moment to let her know that she deserves the support. That sharing food is a beautiful act of community and people want to help. And that this is not just about supporting them when and if they are really struggling, it is also about giving them a chance to feel relaxed and joyful with their newborn.

Encourage her to get really specific about what her family needs and wants. And let her know that if her needs change, you are there to relay the message to her community.

Food: Ask your friends for their family's food allergies, sensitivities, and preferences. From this you can come up with a list of "No foods" and a list of "Yes foods," and even a list of "go light foods". It can also include general guidelines, such as "organic" or "no preservatives" or "nutrient dense". What are some of her favorite dishes? What does she have a hard time digesting? Really, encourage her to be completely honest with this: people want to bring food that she and her family will like and can eat! She can also add easy options for people such as restaurants or deli's she would like take out from and the specific menu choices that she prefers. There are also dinner delivery services -go with the small, local companies.

Something else to discuss with her is common foods that postpartum women avoid. Postpartum food avoidance is cross-cultural, though the foods that are avoided are not. Some commonly avoided foods are beans, onions, garlic, spicy foods, kale, broccoli, citrus, cold foods, chocolate, and caffeine. Some food avoidance is about how the foods affect the baby through the breast milk and others are about the mother's health. If a mother has a hard time with a specific food, it is likely her baby will too.

In planning a postpartum diet parents can look to the traditions of their families as well as the broader wisdom of their cultures of origin. Traditional systems of medicine have specific dietary protocols and dishes for the postpartum time and this some of this knowledge can be found in books, such as the First Forty days by Heng Ou.

These include potent herbal formulas, specific traditional dishes, and a nuanced approach to clearing and warming the uterus. For the sake of brevity, what follows is a much simplified explanation. Central to these practices is the belief that food is a powerful way to balance and restore a postpartum persons's body. Foods are seen as warming, cooling, or neutral based on their principles and affects within the body. Some warming foods include ginger, onions, chicken and squash. Cooling foods are cucumber, lettuce, tofu, and peppermint tea. Postpartum women are especially discouraged from eating frozen, cold, or even raw foods. Broths and well cooked soups are common and are good examples of easily digestible foods -another important principle.

Meal Train Guide

VISITORS: It is so important to set clear boundaries, based on what your friend is wanting. Bringing a meal is not necessarily an invitation to visit. Encourage her not to feel obligated to visit, let people hold the baby or even say hi. This allows her to receive meals from whomever would like to bring food, not just the small circle of people she wants to visit with. Maybe she is private and would like a note on the front door saying "Thank you for the meal. The mother and baby are resting and aren't available for visiting". It can be added that if people are coming in to the house, they need to wash their hands, and if they or someone in their household is sick to cancel the meal delivery. Also you can point out to your friend that she has access to the on line sign up so that she can see who is coming when.

TIME LINE: A good Meal Train can go for a month or even two months. The on line schedule will allow you to choose a span of time and then to go in and take out specific dates. So if a Grandma will be visiting for 10 days during the baby's first month, simply take those dates out -but only if Grandma has specifically agreed to cooking! Maybe the family wants meals for a month solid and then 4 days a week for the second month. Or maybe the meals increase when her partner goes back to work. If unexpected challenges arise with recovery or the baby, add on more time. Encourage your friend to really receive the help, that sharing food is beautiful and what friends are for. She will have plenty of time to share food with others in the future.

DROP OFF: This should include address, time frame (example: 4-6 pm), and where exactly to put the meal. Sometimes a hot meal is left on the door step or the cooks come in for a visit. It can also be delivered cold and put in a cooler on the front porch -this allows for delivery any time of day. If your friend lives in the country, another option is to have a cooler at a drop off site which will then be picked up by a partner or neighbor and delivered later.

CONTAINERS: It is important to give specific directions with this, so that the receiving family doesn't end up with extra work. Here are some options: deliver food in containers that do not need to be returned -yogurt containers or mason jars. For containers that do need to be returned such as bowls and pots, the name of the family can be taped to the bottom and then the container can be left on the front or back porch to be picked up later.

PEOPLE: Ask your friend for the email addresses or phone numbers of her friends and family she knows will want to sign up. You can also ask her for the key people in her circles of friends. Her circles of friends may include her work, her partner's work, church, neighbors, volunteer groups, kids' schools etc.

CREATING THE CIRCLE: Discuss Step two with her.

Meal Train Guide

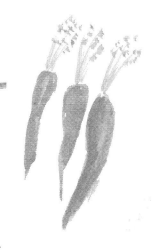

Step 2 create the circle

Initially, it is good to send out an email to the first list of people your friend gives you, let them know what you are up to and give them permission to share this with others. To gather more emails you can contact the key people from your friends' circles and ask them if they can spread the word further. This can also be done later.

Sometimes, it is enough to simply send out a short email to the circle of friends announcing your plan to have a Meal Train for this family. Let them know that you will send out an email when the baby is born. Some circles of friends will jump for the chance to bring a meal and fully understand what it is all about. Other people will need more explanation and encouragement. Maybe they don't do very much home cooking or don't know what a meal Train is or even understand why the family of a newborn would find it so helpful. Here are some ideas about how to stir up excitement about the Meal Train.

At the baby shower or mama blessing:

- Pass around an email sign up on a clip board.
- Give the gift of to go containers or casserole dishes with lids with a card saying "Meal Train."
- Pass out a little card with the sign up site and passwords, with an explanation of the Meal Train.
- Collect frozen dishes at the gathering.

Online:

- Set up a facebook page "The Owen Family Meal Train" and post photos of the baby and updates about the family.
- Set up a Pinterest board "the Owen Family Cook Book" for recipes that will work for the family and give everyone pinning power.

Meal Train Guide

Step 3 activate and keep it coming

Set up the online schedule:
How you need to set up the on line sign up sheet. There are many on line websites for organizing a Meal Train. Choose a site that does not require participants to create an account and sign in. They should only need to give the family's name and password. www.takethemameal.com is what I use, www.mealtrain.com is also good. Once you set up your own account, then set up the family's schedule. Put in the dates and add your cooks instructions to the notes. Setting this up can come before the baby is born and then just adjust the dates as needed.

First email:
The baby is born! Time to activate the Meal Train!
Now is the time to tell folks to start cooking! This can be an email sent BCC to the whole group, announcing the baby's birth and giving all the specifics of the Meal Train and giving the link and password to the on line schedule. Tell people to sign up well in advance, marking down what they will be cooking. The family will be able to see the schedule and it can be helpful for them to see it filled in at least a week or two in advance. People can sign up once or they can sign up once a week for a number of weeks. You can let people know they can simply double their recipe and cook for their own family at the same time, and that simple cooking is appreciated. Even though you have put the cook's notes on the site, go ahead and put them in this email as well.

Follow up emails:
As the coordinator it is your job to check the schedule to make sure it is filling up. You also need to check back with the family to see if any changes are needed or if there is other information that they would like relayed. With follow up emails you can share news about the family (that they wish to share of course), or maybe a photo of the baby. Also include any updates to the cook's instructions. This could be foods she's craving or anything that is not working. And if the schedule is looking empty ask people to sign up again.

When the Meal Train is all finished up, you can send a thank you email out to everyone who participated.

Meal Train Guide

Coordinator's Notes ~for making the cook's instructions~

- Family member names
- Address
- Phone number
- Email

Yes Foods

No Foods

Go Light Foods

Take Out Meals

Time Line

Drop Off

Containers

Visitors Instructions

Discussion about creating the circle

Meal Train Sign-Up

Name	Email	Phone

Congratulations!

You gave birth to your baby and your family has come through those early days, weeks, and months. You have found your way.

You did it!!!

Now you can spread this love and support in your community.

Gratitude

There is a big circle of support around this workbook with so many people to thank.
Alesha Adamson, Silke Akerson, Mitch Bacon, Marissa Bolaños, Sejal Fichadia, Carol Gray, Sara Hart, Stephanie Johne, Courtney Jarecki, Emberlyn Kelly, Kellie Latona, Sister MorningStar, Mirra Nerrenberg, Tiffany Nguyen, Rebeckah Orton, Kate Parks, Elisabeth Pietila, Katerina Perkhova, Amanda Roe, Jennie Sharp, Erin Sweeny, Iris Sullivan, Janet Weidman and many more. Thank you.

Thank you to the many mothers who have shared their experiences with me and given me feedback on the workbook process.

And I am grateful for the love and support of my family.

About Kestrel Gates

Kestrel Gates is a homeschooling mother of two who lives on the Oregon coast. She is passionate about reclaiming postpartum as a time of deep recovery and sweet bonding, a time of strengthening communities, a time when mothering and parenting are valued and celebrated.

Please email any questions or feedback to: kestrel@buildyournestworkbook.com
And if you loved the workbook, please review it on Amazon!

Bulk orders available at: www.buildyournestworkbook.com

For Parents

Start a BYN Book Club
buildyournestworkbook.com/book-club-kit

Find a Postpartum Navigator
buildyournestworkbook.com/postpartum-navigators-directory

Download Free Resources
buildyournestworkbook.com/free-online-resources

For Professionals

BYN Book Club Kit
buildyournestworkbook.com/book-club-kit

Postpartum Navigator Training
buildyournestworkbook.com/navigator-training

All the BYN Free Resources
https://rb.gy/717ez

Monthly Workbook Subscription
shop.buildyournestworkbook.com

Buy a 10 Pack of Workbooks
shop.buildyournestworkbook.com

Made in the USA
Monee, IL
27 June 2023

37724067R00059